Nonprescription Drugs in Pregnancy

Your Guide to Fetal Risk for the Active Ingredients in 500 Over-The-Counter Drugs

by

D. Gary Benfield, M.D.

Smart Start Press

To purchase copies of *Nonprescription Drugs in Pregnancy*,
use any of the following ways:

Go to www.atlasbooks.com

Phone: 800-247-6553

Fax: 419-281-6883

or

Order from your favorite bookstore

Copyright 2010, D. Gary Benfield, M.D.
Smart Start Press

ISBN: 978-0-9779848-7-9

LCCN: 2010916797

The information contained in this book is not intended to substitute for your own doctor's medical advice. Readers should always consult their doctors or other healthcare providers for advice and treatment. If you are pregnant or planning a pregnancy, always let your doctor know before taking any drug, prescription or nonprescription, or herbal remedy. The author and the publisher disclaim any liability arising directly or indirectly from the use of this book.

The purpose of providing some 500 nonprescription drug examples is to reflect the use of active ingredients rather than providing an inclusive list of all brands on the market. The sources used to identify the randomly selected sample are listed in the Appendix under References. The inclusion of a brand name does not mean the author or the publisher has any particular knowledge that the brand listed has any particular properties different from other brands of the same drug, nor should it be interpreted as an endorsement by the author or the publisher. Similarly, the fact that a particular brand has not been included does not indicate that the drug has been judged to be unsatisfactory or unacceptable. Furthermore, the use of a brand name in this book is not intended as a grant of authority to exercise any right or privilege protected by a patent or trademark owned by the drug's manufacturer. Registered trademarks for the nonprescription drugs listed in this book are located in the Appendix.

All rights reserved. No part of this book may be reproduced or transmitted in any form or by any means, electronic or mechanical, including photocopying, recording, or by information storage and retrieval systems, without the written permission of the publisher, except by a reviewer who may quote brief passages in a review.

Printed in the United States of America.

Table of Contents

I	Foreword	v
II	Introduction	ix
III	Acknowledgments	xiii
IV	Reading a Nonprescription Drug Label	xv
V	FDA Pregnancy Risk Categories (A, B, C, D, X) for the Active Ingredients in Nonprescription Drugs	xviii
VI	How to Use This Book	xxi
VII	Pregnancy Risk Profiles for the Active Ingredients in 500 Nonprescription Drugs, Divided into 14 Clinical Sections:	1

1. Allergy, Sinus & Asthma   *2*
2. Cold, Cough & Flu   *39*
3. Constipation   *118*
4. Diarrhea   *134*
5. Fungal, Yeast and Other Infections   *142*
6. Gas   *151*
7. Heartburn & Reflux Disease   *160*
8. Menstrual Discomfort   *190*
9. Motion Sickness   *198*
10. Pain Relief & Fever Reduction   *205*
11. Skin Disorders   *257*
12. Sleep Aids   *276*

13. Smoking Aids *287*
14. The Remainder *292*

VIII A Three-Step Process for Creating a Pregnancy Risk Profile of the Active Ingredients in a Nonprescription Drug© 296

IX Appendix
1. Non-Steroidal, Anti-Inflammatory Drugs (NSAIDS) in Pregnancy *305*
2. Taking Acetaminophen: The Good and the Ugly *307*
3. References *311*
4. Trademarks for the Over-The-Counter Drugs in This Book *313*

X Index of 500 Over-The-Counter Drugs in This Book 318

Foreword

I want to thank Dr. Benfield, the author, for the opportunity to read and comment on this unique book before anyone else got the chance. What a treat! Since I'm a family doctor, who also practices obstetrics, and I'm the mother of four young daughters, I read this book from several perspectives. And while reading, I also heard my father's voice since he wrote the book.

Even as a physician, I have to admit that I often feel overwhelmed sorting through the seemingly endless array of brightly colored bottles, boxes and tubes of over-the-counter medicines lining the shelves at the drugstore. And if I feel overwhelmed, you can only imagine what a sleep-deprived pregnant woman, also suffering from heartburn, might feel as she too sorts through the endless array for a sleep aid and an acid reducer while wondering what she's going to fix for supper. Hey! I've been there and done that.

Now, along comes this remarkable book, one that no one else has written.

- First, we find what the author calls "A Pregnancy Risk Profile" of the active ingredients in each of some 500 over-the-counter drugs (A pregnancy risk profile is a list of the active ingredients, typically one to five, in each drug and their pregnancy risk categories, A, B, C, or D; no X's). The possibility that a pregnant woman might relax with this book in the comfort of her own home and locate one or more over-the-counter drugs with the safest active ingredients to treat her symptoms has the potential to be a significant and innovative advance in healthcare for pregnant women. And if you are a pharmacist, nurse, doctor, or student training to become one of these professionals, the book will be a valuable resource for you too. After all, it's you that most pregnant women turn to for this kind of advice.

- Second, the book offers a simple "Three-Step Process for Creating a Pregnancy Risk Profile of the Active Ingredients in a Nonprescription Drug©" for over-the-counter drugs not found in the book.
- Third, the book contains other treasures, such as a section on how to read a nonprescription drug label, called Drug Facts; a section that spells out how to use the book; and a section that explains each of the FDA's Five Pregnancy Risk Categories: A, B, C, D, X. Of course, there are no category X (highest risk) active ingredients in over-the-counter drugs.

Shortly before reading this book, a pregnant woman came to see me for congestion and facial pressure. I diagnosed her with a sinus infection. When she asked what over-the-counter drug she could take to help relieve her symptoms, I could only think of one active ingredient. But, even then, I couldn't direct her to the brand name drugs that contain this active ingredient. So I effectively sent her on a scavenger hunt to the drugstore, hoping she could find the right drug.

Soon after I read this book, I encountered a similar scenario with another patient. Only this time my response was different. To relieve her symptoms, I suggested she try Tylenol® Cold Head Congestion Daytime, containing acetaminophen (Pregnancy risk category B); dextromethorphan (Pregnancy risk category C); and phenylephrine (Pregnancy risk category C). On the other hand, if she preferred a liquid, she could take Theraflu® Warming Relief Daytime Severe Cold, which contains the same active ingredients. Since cost was an issue for this patient, it felt good to be able to offer her the names of several products, each containing the same active ingredients, but selling for different prices. As for my patient, she headed out to the drugstore armed with my recommendations, empowered to choose the product that not only fit her illness and her desire for fetal safety, but her budget as well.

Clearly, as a physician, this book is going to be an immense help to me and my colleagues in the clinic, including our triage nurse who will have her own personal copy.

But what I really like about this book is what it will do for pregnant women. It empowers them to make well-informed decisions about

Foreword

over-the-counter medicines they may choose to take. But the book also contains the following reminder after each drug entry: "If you are pregnant or planning a pregnancy, always let your healthcare provider know before taking any drug, prescription or nonprescription, or herbal remedy." Armed with the information in this book, those conversations with your healthcare provider should be less intimidating and more rewarding than ever before. After all, you'll be closer to speaking the same language.

When my dad told me about a year ago that he was going to write this book, I couldn't wait to get my hands on it. I don't know how many times I told the family practice residents I teach, "Soon, we are going to have a book that will help us with this," as we clicked through Web sites searching for the most appropriate over-the-counter cold preparations and constipation remedies for our pregnant patients. I am thrilled that day has arrived, for now we have a quick, concise yet thorough reference to help us help our pregnant patients. And for those pregnant women and their families reading this, now you have a tool that will help you talk with your healthcare provider about what medicines are safe to take in pregnancy.

So here's to a happy, healthy pregnancy. And, should you have some aches and pains along the way, hopefully this book will bring you comfort.

Introduction

Nonprescription drugs are commonly known as over-the-counter drugs or OTC drugs. They are sold in pharmacies, grocery stores, convenience stores, mass retail outlets, and over the Internet, enabling consumers to self-diagnose and self-treat certain ailments without consulting a physician.[1]

Many women who are planning their pregnancies or already pregnant buy OTC drugs for a variety of symptoms and illnesses, including seasonal allergy, sinus and asthma; cold, cough and flu; constipation; diarrhea; fungal, yeast, and other infections; gas; heartburn; motion sickness; pain relief and fever reduction; skin disorders; difficulty sleeping; and smoking cessation. These women are eager to know if OTC drugs are safe for unborn babies. The following true story illustrates their concern:

In the spring of 2010, a pregnant lady asked our local pharmacist if it was safe to take Benadryl for her allergies. The pharmacist knew the active ingredient in Benadryl is diphenhydramine, an antihistamine. The pharmacist also knew that what the woman was really asking is diphenhydramine, the active ingredient, safe for her baby? But the pharmacist couldn't remember what pregnancy risk category (A, B, C, D, or X) diphenhydramine belonged to, and she didn't have a source to look it up. So she told the woman she thought Benadryl was safe, but she should check with her doctor first. The pharmacist felt somewhat uneasy saying this, because she knew most doctors in the area were not familiar with the active ingredients in over-the-counter drugs or their pregnancy risk categories.

The following day, the pharmacist happened to share this story with me, the author. I asked her if it would help to have that kind of information all in one place, such as in a book. "I'd buy that book in a minute," she said. "I get calls all the time from doctors' offices and pregnant women wanting to know if this or that drug is safe to take in pregnancy. They don't put that kind of information about active ingredients on over-the-counter drugs."

The idea for this book was conceived at that moment. If what my pharmacist had said was true, such a book would not only help pregnant women, it would also help pharmacists, doctors, nurses, and students too.

The core of this book is found in Part VII, which contains the pregnancy risk categories (A, B, C, D, X) for the active ingredients in more than 500 over-the-counter drugs. We call them pregnancy risk profiles. If, however, you have a nonprescription drug in mind that's not in this book, Part VIII shows you how to create your own pregnancy risk profile using our easy-to-follow, three-step process.

Now, what is an active ingredient? An active ingredient is actually a drug that treats the patient's symptoms. Over-the-counter drugs typically contain from one to five active ingredients. But when the patient is pregnant, most active ingredients cross the placenta, enter the fetal bloodstream, and "treat" the fetus too. So whenever a pregnant woman uses almost any drug, prescription or nonprescription, or herbal remedy, she is taking the drug for two.

Let's repeat: nonprescription drugs contain one to five active ingredients, which are actually drugs themselves. For example, the number of active ingredients in the 521 nonprescription drugs profiled in Part VII break down like this:

- One active ingredient – 253 drugs (48.6%)
- Two active ingredients – 122 drugs (23.4%)
- Three active ingredients – 118 drugs (22.6%)
- Four active ingredients – 27 drugs (5.2%)
- Five active ingredients – 1 drug (0.2%)

Introducing the "Rx-to-OTC Switch"[2]

Twenty to thirty years ago, many of those active ingredients were actually FDA-approved prescription drugs. As prescription drugs, they were assigned a pregnancy risk category: A, B, C, D, or X. As time

Introduction

passed and those drugs established a track record of safety and effectiveness, their manufacturers obtained FDA approval for the "Rx-to-OTC switch," meaning they could be sold over-the-counter as active ingredients in nonprescription drugs. And their pregnancy risk categories still applied.

For example, prior to 1981, diphenhydramine, the antihistamine we met earlier in the Benadryl story, was a prescription drug with a pregnancy risk category of **B**.[3] In 1981, the drug was first approved for over-the-counter use as an active ingredient in Benylin®, a cough medicine. The following year, diphenhydramine's tendency to cause drowsiness was put to use as the active ingredient in Sominex®, a sleep aid. That same year, it was also included as an active ingredient in Excedrin PM®, another sleep aid. In 1985, diphenhydramine was approved as the active ingredient in Benadryl®, an over-the-counter allergy medicine. In 1987, diphenhydramine was approved for over-the-counter sale as an active ingredient in drugs for motion sickness. More recently, diphenhydramine was approved in 2005 as an active ingredient in Advil PM®, an analgesic sleep aid. So you see, thanks to the Rx-to-OTC switch, diphenhydramine is found in numerous OTC drugs, which are used for a variety of clinical purposes, while retaining its pregnancy risk category of B.

Now we can begin to understand why the FDA does not assign an overall pregnancy risk category to each nonprescription drug. Instead, the FDA relies on the pregnancy risk category of each active ingredient as an indicator of fetal safety. However, since this information does not appear on an OTC drug's label, called "Drug Facts," this book is designed to help fill this need.

Introducing the "OTC-to-Rx Switch"

As we said earlier in the introduction, when a pregnant woman takes an OTC drug, its active ingredients are absorbed into her bloodstream, typically cross the placenta, and "treat" the fetus too. So she is raising the risk by taking the drug for two: one adult and one rapidly developing fetus whose ability to metabolize the active ingredients is still developing too.

Most OTC Drug Facts labels say consult your physician before taking this drug if you are pregnant. In effect, the drug maker is saying, "Before you raise the risk by taking this drug for two, we want you, the pregnant consumer, to reverse the Rx-to-OTC switch (which enables consumers to self-diagnose and self-treat their ailments without seeing a doctor) and undergo an OTC-to-Rx switch, meaning regard this OTC drug as a prescription drug and seek your doctor's advice."

This book also contains other handy and helpful parts:

- Part IV – Reading a Nonprescription Drug Label
- Part VI – How to Use This Book
- Appendix:
    - Non-Steroidal, Anti-Inflammatory Drugs (NSAIDs) in Pregnancy
    - Taking Acetaminophen: The Good and the Ugly
- Part X – Index of 500 Over-The-Counter Drugs in This Book

Don't miss them.

Acknowledgments

This book is dedicated with loving affection to the devoted staff of the Neonatal Intensive Care Unit at Akron Children's Hospital, Akron, Ohio and to the memory of Jane Nichols, pioneering Head of Bereavement Services at Akron Children's, who taught us how to care for dying and newly deceased children and their grieving parents. Amen.

* * * *

Thank you, Malia Lane, for your typing and organizational skills; Ryan Feasel for creating the cover; and Cynthia Kelley, D.O. for writing the Foreword.

D. Gary Benfield, M.D.

Reading a Nonprescription Drug Label

The Food and Drug Administration (FDA) requires that all drugs sold over-the-counter have an eight-item drug label called "Drug Facts."[4] The eight items are always listed in the same order to help consumers choose the right medication to treat their symptoms, use the medication correctly, and get the most benefit from the drug. Let's list the eight items, then discuss them one by one:

- Active ingredient(s)
- Purpose for each active ingredient
- Uses
- Warnings
- Directions
- Other information
- Inactive ingredients
- Questions

Active Ingredient(s)

As we learned in the introduction, over-the-counter drugs contain from one to five active ingredients, which are actually drugs themselves. Their purpose is to treat the patient's symptoms. But when the patient is pregnant, the active ingredients typically cross the placenta, enter the fetal bloodstream, and "treat" the fetus too. So whenever a pregnant woman uses any drug, prescription or nonprescription, or herbal remedy, she is taking the drug for two.

Once a pregnant woman or her clinician have identified the active ingredient(s) by reading the first item in Drug Facts, they can simply turn to Section VIII in this book, look up the active ingredient(s) and identify their pregnancy risk categories: A, B, C, D, or X. (By the way, there are no Category X active ingredients in OTC drugs.) Armed with this information, she and her clinician will be in a better position to decide if the potential benefit of taking the drug is greater than the potential risk for unborn babies.

Also, if a pregnant woman is taking more than one drug, knowledge of the active ingredients in whatever drugs she's taking will minimize the risk of her taking too much of the same active ingredient and harming herself or her unborn baby. (See "Taking Acetaminophen: The Good and the Ugly" in the Appendix for the case example of a pregnant woman who exceeded the safe daily limit of 4,000 mg of acetaminophen when she inadvertently took two drugs that both contained acetaminophen.)

Active Ingredient Purpose

This section tells you what the purpose of each active ingredient is, such as an antihistamine or a laxative.

Uses

This section explains the symptoms for which the drug should be used. You should only use a drug that's designed to treat your symptoms. If pregnant, this decision should be shared with your clinician.

Warnings

There are times when you should not take a particular OTC drug. For example, if you are allergic to one of its active ingredients. That warning appears in this section. You will be warned in this section to consult your physician or another healthcare professional if you are pregnant or breastfeeding. Potential side effects are also listed here and what to do if you experience them.

Reading a Nonprescription Drug Label **xvii**

This section usually includes a warning to KEEP THIS DRUG OUT OF REACH OF CHILDREN and what to do in case of an overdose.

Directions

This section tells you how much, how often, and for how long to take a drug. It's just as important to follow these instructions for an OTC drug as it is for a prescription drug.

Other Information

This section contains information about storing the drug and other tidbits that don't fit under other headings.

Inactive Ingredients

This section may include important information if you or a family member happen to be allergic to one of these inactive ingredients.

Questions

This section advises you to contact your pharmacist, doctor, or other healthcare professional if you have questions.

The FDA's Pregnancy Risk Categories: A, B, C, D, X

Adapted to the Active Ingredients in Nonprescription Drugs

Category A: Controlled studies using the active ingredient in pregnant women have not shown harmful fetal effects throughout pregnancy, and the possibility of fetal harm seems remote. My comment: *Though apparently safe, these active ingredients should still only be used in pregnancy when clearly indicated.*

Category B: Either studies have shown no evidence of fetal harm when using the active ingredient in pregnant animals, but no controlled studies have been done in pregnant women, **or** studies have shown evidence of fetal harm when using the active ingredient in pregnant animals, but controlled studies in pregnant women have not shown evidence of fetal harm. My comment: *These active ingredients should only be used in pregnancy when clearly indicated.*

Category C: Either studies have shown evidence of fetal harm when using the active ingredient in pregnant animals, but no controlled studies have been done in pregnant women, **or** studies using the active ingredient in pregnant animals have not been done, and studies of pregnant women are insufficient to reach a conclusion. These active ingredients should only be used by a pregnant woman if the potential

The FDA's Pregnancy Risk Categories xix

benefit justifies the potential risk of fetal harm, which, in many cases, is unknown. My comment: *It's impossible to calculate the potential risk of fetal harm when, in many cases, it's unknown. Thus, these active ingredients should only be used in pregnancy when clearly needed.*

Category D: Studies have shown evidence of fetal harm when using the active ingredient in pregnant women. However, the potential benefit of using the active ingredient in some life-threatening situations for mom may outweigh the potential risk of fetal harm. For example, when mom requires cancer treatment or when she has a serious disease for which safer active ingredients cannot be used or are less effective. My comment: *These exceptional indications rarely occur when considering a nonprescription drug in pregnancy.*

Category X: My comment: *Because the risk of fetal harm is too high, no Category X active ingredients have been approved for use in nonprescription drugs.*

Active Ingredients Assigned Two Pregnancy Risk Categories: Some active ingredients have two pregnancy risk categories, depending on which trimester of pregnancy the active ingredient is used. For example, naproxen sodium, the active ingredient in Aleve, belongs to Category **B** when used in the first and second trimesters of pregnancy. If used in the third trimester, however, the active ingredient belongs to Category **D**. My comment: *This means naproxen sodium should not be used in the third trimester unless prescribed by a physician who has advised her patient of the risks involved.*[5]

Notes

1. As mentioned in the Introduction, the active ingredients in nonprescription drugs are actually drugs themselves. Many were once prescription drugs – some 20 to 30 years ago – when they were assigned by the FDA to a Pregnancy Risk Category: A, B, C, D, or X. Even though these drugs were eventually approved to switch from prescription to nonprescription status and sold over-the-counter (OTC) as active ingredients, their original pregnancy risk categories still apply.

2. There are seven Category **D** active ingredients among the 521 nonprescription drugs found in this book. Three of them – aspirin, ibuprofen, and naproxen sodium – are non-steroidal, anti-inflammatory drugs, or NSAIDs. They are Category **D** only if used in the third trimester of pregnancy. Of the four remaining active ingredients, hydrocortisone is Category **D** if used in the first trimester; Codeine phosphate is Category **D** if used for prolonged periods in pregnancy or in high doses near term; and Povidone-Iodine, 10% and Nicotine are both Category **D** throughout pregnancy.

3. **The FDA's New Proposal to Eliminate the Current Pregnancy Risk Categories A, B, C, D, X.** In 2008, the FDA proposed a new rule to eliminate the current Pregnancy Risk Categories A, B, C, D, X in favor of a more informative method of labeling prescription drugs for pregnancy and lactation.[6] One of the concerns was that the five Categories A, B, C, D, X might mislead healthcare providers and the women they counsel into believing that fetal risk simply increases from Category A to B to C to D to X. This may oversimplify the process of weighing potential fetal harm versus potential maternal benefit, especially for drugs that fall in Category **C**.

Unfortunately, the information needed from drug studies in pregnant animals and in pregnant women for estimating potential fetal harm is often woefully inadequate. That's unlikely to change much, regardless of which method the FDA endorses for labeling prescription drugs in the future.

Based on the FDA's progress to date, the sweeping changes proposed in its new rule may take several more years before they are published in final form. After that, it will likely take five to ten years to fully implement those changes, according to the timetable outlined in the proposal. Meanwhile, you can count on this handy guide to help answer your questions about fetal risk. And when the time comes, a revised edition will keep you up-to-date.

How to Use This Book

There are three easy ways for expectant moms and clinicians to use this book:

1. **By Symptom**: Let's say you want to find the Pregnancy Risk Profile for a particular nonprescription drug used to treat constipation. You open the book to Part VII where more than 500 over-the-counter drugs are organized into 14 clinical sections. You turn to Constipation, which is Section 3. You find the drug you have in mind, Dulcolax® Stool Softener. The drug's Pregnancy Risk Profile reveals a single active ingredient, docusate sodium. Its pregnancy risk category is C. You then turn to the end of the section for an explanation of all the pregnancy risk categories, including category C.

    The explanation for category C is not very reassuring. So you browse through Section 3, looking for other alternatives. You discover the Pregnancy Risk Profile for the active ingredient(s) in Metamucil® Fiber Laxative. It also has a single active ingredient (psyllium husk), but its pregnancy risk category is B. That may be a safer choice, but since you are four months pregnant and have a doctor's appointment tomorrow, you decide to take the book with you and discuss the decision of which drug to buy with your doctor first.

2. **By Brand Name**: Since you were looking for a particular brand name at first, you could have gone directly to Part X, "Index of 500 Over-The-Counter Drugs in This Book," and found Dulcolax® Stool Softener that way.

3. **For Unlisted Drugs**: Suppose the nonprescription drug you are interested in is not listed in this book. You can easily create your own Pregnancy Risk Profile for the active ingredient(s) in the drug of interest by turning to Part VIII, "A Three-Step Process for Creating a Pregnancy Risk Profile of the Active Ingredients in a Nonprescription Drug."© Here's the three-step process in a nutshell:

Step 1 – Identify the active ingredient(s) in the drug of interest. This is the first item on the drug label called Drug Facts. (See Part IV, "Reading a Nonprescription Drug Label," for more details.)

Step 2 – Identify the pregnancy risk category: A, B, C, D, X for each active ingredient in the drug of interest by turning to the table at the end of Part VIII, "Table of Active Ingredients and Their Pregnancy Risk Categories." Note: There are no Category X active ingredients in nonprescription drugs.

Step 3 – Turn to Part V or the end of any section for an explanation of each pregnancy risk category found in Step 2.

Your Pregnancy Risk Profile is now complete, including an explanation for the pregnancy risk category of each active ingredient.

Additional Tips

1. Be sure to read the Introduction if you haven't done so already. It contains information about nonprescription drugs that may be unfamiliar to many doctors, nurses, and pregnant women while introducing you in a practical way to the rest of this book. It's time well spent.

2. Don't forget to read the first two articles in Part IX, "Appendix." Pregnant or not, the article "Taking Acetaminophen: The Good and The Ugly" contains useful information every consumer and healthcare provider should know. Most folks are unaware that even though acetaminophen is the pain reliever/fever reducer of choice in pregnancy, it's also the number one cause of acute liver failure in this country when used incorrectly.[7]

Pregnancy Risk Profiles for the Active Ingredients in 500 Nonprescription Drugs

Section 1: Allergy, Sinus & Asthma

Actifed® Cold & Allergy Tablets

Active Ingredient:	Pregnancy Risk Category:
Chlorpheniramine maleate	B
Phenylephrine Hcl	C

Helpful Hints and Reminders: Each pregnancy risk category (**A**, **B**, **C**, **D**, or **X**) is explained on the last page of this section.

Remember: All pregnancies have a background risk of 3% or more for a serious birth defect, even when mom doesn't take a drug of any kind. If you are pregnant or planning a pregnancy, always let your healthcare provider know before taking any drug, prescription or non-prescription, or herbal remedy.

Advil® Allergy Sinus Caplets

Active Ingredient:	Pregnancy Risk Category:
Chlorpheniramine maleate	B
Pseudoephedrine Hcl	C

(continued)

Ibuprofen	Ibuprofen has two pregnancy risk categories: **B** when used in the first or second trimesters of pregnancy; **D** if used in the third trimester. (See Helpful Hints below.)

Helpful Hints and Reminders: Each pregnancy risk category (**A**, **B**, **C**, **D**, or **X**) is explained on the last page of this section.

1. Ibuprofen is a member of the non-steroidal, anti-inflammatory family of drugs, or NSAIDs. Members of this family of drugs should not be used during the third trimester of pregnancy (last 12 weeks) unless specifically prescribed by a clinician. See the Appendix for "Non-Steroidal, Anti-Inflammatory Drugs (NSAIDs) in Pregnancy," which describes the serious problems these drugs may cause for unborn babies when taken in the third trimester of pregnancy.

2. Women attempting to conceive should not use any NSAID, including Ibuprofen, because of the findings in animals that these drugs may block implantation of the early embryo in the wall of the uterus, in effect preventing pregnancy.

Remember: All pregnancies have a background risk of 3% or more for a serious birth defect, even when mom doesn't take a drug of any kind. If you are pregnant or planning a pregnancy, always let your healthcare provider know before taking any drug, prescription or non-prescription, or herbal remedy.

Afrin® 12 Hour Spray, Sinus

Active Ingredient:	Pregnancy Risk Category:
Oxymetazoline hydrochloride	C

Helpful Hints and Reminders: Each pregnancy risk category (**A**, **B**, **C**, **D**, or **X**) is explained on the last page of this section.

Remember: All pregnancies have a background risk of 3% or more for a serious birth defect, even when mom doesn't take a drug of any kind.

If you are pregnant or planning a pregnancy, always let your healthcare provider know before taking any drug, prescription or non-prescription, or herbal remedy.

Afrin® All Night No Drip, Nasal Spray

Active Ingredient:	Pregnancy Risk Category:
Oxymetazoline hydrochloride	C

Helpful Hints and Reminders: Each pregnancy risk category (**A**, **B**, **C**, **D**, or **X**) is explained on the last page of this section.

Remember: All pregnancies have a background risk of 3% or more for a serious birth defect, even when mom doesn't take a drug of any kind. If you are pregnant or planning a pregnancy, always let your healthcare provider know before taking any drug, prescription or non-prescription, or herbal remedy.

Afrin® No Drip Original 12 Hour Pump Mist, Extra Moisturizing

Active Ingredient:	Pregnancy Risk Category:
Oxymetazoline hydrochloride	C

Helpful Hints and Reminders: Each pregnancy risk category (**A**, **B**, **C**, **D**, or **X**) is explained on the last page of this section.

Remember: All pregnancies have a background risk of 3% or more for a serious birth defect, even when mom doesn't take a drug of any kind. If you are pregnant or planning a pregnancy, always let your healthcare provider know before taking any drug, prescription or non-prescription, or herbal remedy.

Afrin® No Drip 12 Hour Pump Mist, Severe Congestion

Active Ingredient:	Pregnancy Risk Category:
Oxymetazoline hydrochloride	C

Helpful Hints and Reminders: Each pregnancy risk category (**A**, **B**, **C**, **D**, or **X**) is explained on the last page of this section.

Remember: All pregnancies have a background risk of 3% or more for a serious birth defect, even when mom doesn't take a drug of any kind. If you are pregnant or planning a pregnancy, always let your healthcare provider know before taking any drug, prescription or non-prescription, or herbal remedy.

Afrin® No Drip Original 12 Hour Pump Mist

Active Ingredient:	Pregnancy Risk Category:
Oxymetazoline hydrochloride	C

Helpful Hints and Reminders: Each pregnancy risk category (**A**, **B**, **C**, **D**, or **X**) is explained on the last page of this section.

Remember: All pregnancies have a background risk of 3% or more for a serious birth defect, even when mom doesn't take a drug of any kind. If you are pregnant or planning a pregnancy, always let your healthcare provider know before taking any drug, prescription or non-prescription, or herbal remedy.

Alavert® Allergy & Sinus D-12 Hour Tablets

Active Ingredient:	Pregnancy Risk Category:
Loratadine	B
Pseudoephedrine	C

Helpful Hints and Reminders: Each pregnancy risk category (**A**, **B**, **C**, **D**, or **X**) is explained on the last page of this section.

Remember: All pregnancies have a background risk of 3% or more for a serious birth defect, even when mom doesn't take a drug of any kind. If you are pregnant or planning a pregnancy, always let your healthcare provider know before taking any drug, prescription or non-prescription, or herbal remedy.

Alavert® Tablets

Active Ingredient:	Pregnancy Risk Category:
Loratadine	B

Helpful Hints and Reminders: Each pregnancy risk category (**A**, **B**, **C**, **D**, or **X**) is explained on the last page of this section.

Remember: All pregnancies have a background risk of 3% or more for a serious birth defect, even when mom doesn't take a drug of any kind. If you are pregnant or planning a pregnancy, always let your healthcare provider know before taking any drug, prescription or non-prescription, or herbal remedy.

Allerest® PE Allergy & Sinus Relief Tablets

Active Ingredient:	Pregnancy Risk Category:
Chlorpheniramine maleate	B
Phenylephrine Hcl	C

Helpful Hints and Reminders: Each pregnancy risk category (**A**, **B**, **C**, **D**, or **X**) is explained on the last page of this section.

Remember: All pregnancies have a background risk of 3% or more for a serious birth defect, even when mom doesn't take a drug of any kind. If you are pregnant or planning a pregnancy, always let your healthcare provider know before taking any drug, prescription or non-prescription, or herbal remedy.

Benadryl® Allergy Kapgels

Active Ingredient:	Pregnancy Risk Category:
Diphenhydramine Hcl	B

Helpful Hints and Reminders: Each pregnancy risk category (**A**, **B**, **C**, **D**, or **X**) is explained on the last page of this section.

Remember: All pregnancies have a background risk of 3% or more for a serious birth defect, even when mom doesn't take a drug of any kind.

If you are pregnant or planning a pregnancy, always let your healthcare provider know before taking any drug, prescription or non-prescription, or herbal remedy.

Benadryl® Allergy Quick Dissolve Strips

Active Ingredient:	Pregnancy Risk Category:
Diphenhydramine Hcl	B

Helpful Hints and Reminders: Each pregnancy risk category (**A**, **B**, **C**, **D**, or **X**) is explained on the last page of this section.

Remember: All pregnancies have a background risk of 3% or more for a serious birth defect, even when mom doesn't take a drug of any kind. If you are pregnant or planning a pregnancy, always let your healthcare provider know before taking any drug, prescription or non-prescription, or herbal remedy.

Benadryl® Allergy Ultratab™ Tablets

Active Ingredient:	Pregnancy Risk Category:
Diphenhydramine Hcl	B

Helpful Hints and Reminders: Each pregnancy risk category (**A**, **B**, **C**, **D**, or **X**) is explained on the last page of this section.

Remember: All pregnancies have a background risk of 3% or more for a serious birth defect, even when mom doesn't take a drug of any kind. If you are pregnant or planning a pregnancy, always let your healthcare provider know before taking any drug, prescription or non-prescription, or herbal remedy.

Benadryl® Dye-Free Allergy Liqui-Gels

Active Ingredient:	Pregnancy Risk Category:
Diphenhydramine Hcl	B

Helpful Hints and Reminders: Each pregnancy risk category (**A**, **B**, **C**, **D**, or **X**) is explained on the last page of this section.

Remember: All pregnancies have a background risk of 3% or more for a serious birth defect, even when mom doesn't take a drug of any kind. If you are pregnant or planning a pregnancy, always let your healthcare provider know before taking any drug, prescription or non-prescription, or herbal remedy.

Benadryl-D® Allergy Plus Sinus

Active Ingredient:	Pregnancy Risk Category:
Diphenhydramine Hcl	B
Phenylephrine Hcl	C

Helpful Hints and Reminders: Each pregnancy risk category (**A**, **B**, **C**, **D**, or **X**) is explained on the last page of this section.

Remember: All pregnancies have a background risk of 3% or more for a serious birth defect, even when mom doesn't take a drug of any kind. If you are pregnant or planning a pregnancy, always let your healthcare provider know before taking any drug, prescription or non-prescription, or herbal remedy.

Chlor-Trimeton® Allergy Relief, 4 Hour Tablets

Active Ingredient:	Pregnancy Risk Category:
Chlorpheniramine maleate	B

Helpful Hints and Reminders: Each pregnancy risk category (**A**, **B**, **C**, **D**, or **X**) is explained on the last page of this section.

Remember: All pregnancies have a background risk of 3% or more for a serious birth defect, even when mom doesn't take a drug of any kind. If you are pregnant or planning a pregnancy, always let your healthcare provider know before taking any drug, prescription or non-prescription, or herbal remedy.

Chlor-Trimeton® Allergy Relief, 12 Hour Tablets

Active Ingredient:	Pregnancy Risk Category:
Chlorpheniramine maleate	B

Helpful Hints and Reminders: Each pregnancy risk category (**A**, **B**, **C**, **D**, or **X**) is explained on the last page of this section.

Remember: All pregnancies have a background risk of 3% or more for a serious birth defect, even when mom doesn't take a drug of any kind. If you are pregnant or planning a pregnancy, always let your healthcare provider know before taking any drug, prescription or non-prescription, or herbal remedy.

Claritin® 12 Hour/24 Hour Non-Drowsy Reditabs®

Active Ingredient:	Pregnancy Risk Category:
Loratadine	B

Helpful Hints and Reminders: Each pregnancy risk category (**A**, **B**, **C**, **D**, or **X**) is explained on the last page of this section.

Remember: All pregnancies have a background risk of 3% or more for a serious birth defect, even when mom doesn't take a drug of any kind. If you are pregnant or planning a pregnancy, always let your healthcare provider know before taking any drug, prescription or non-prescription, or herbal remedy.

Claritin® 24 Hour Non-Drowsy Liqui-Gels

Active Ingredient:	Pregnancy Risk Category:
Loratadine	B

Helpful Hints and Reminders: Each pregnancy risk category (**A**, **B**, **C**, **D**, or **X**) is explained on the last page of this section.

Remember: All pregnancies have a background risk of 3% or more for a serious birth defect, even when mom doesn't take a drug of any kind.

If you are pregnant or planning a pregnancy, always let your healthcare provider know before taking any drug, prescription or non-prescription, or herbal remedy.

Claritin® Eye Itch Relief

Active Ingredient:	Pregnancy Risk Category:
Ketotifen	C

Helpful Hints and Reminders: Each pregnancy risk category (**A**, **B**, **C**, **D**, or **X**) is explained on the last page of this section.

Remember: All pregnancies have a background risk of 3% or more for a serious birth defect, even when mom doesn't take a drug of any kind. If you are pregnant or planning a pregnancy, always let your healthcare provider know before taking any drug, prescription or non-prescription, or herbal remedy.

Claritin® Non-Drowsy Tablets

Active Ingredient:	Pregnancy Risk Category:
Loratadine	B

Helpful Hints and Reminders: Each pregnancy risk category (**A**, **B**, **C**, **D**, or **X**) is explained on the last page of this section.

Remember: All pregnancies have a background risk of 3% or more for a serious birth defect, even when mom doesn't take a drug of any kind. If you are pregnant or planning a pregnancy, always let your healthcare provider know before taking any drug, prescription or non-prescription, or herbal remedy.

Claritin-D® 12 Hour & 24 Hour Non-Drowsy Tablets

Active Ingredient:	Pregnancy Risk Category:
Loratadine	B
Pseudoephedrine	C

DayQuil® Sinus LiquiCaps **11**

Helpful Hints and Reminders: Each pregnancy risk category (**A**, **B**, **C**, **D**, or **X**) is explained on the last page of this section.

Remember: All pregnancies have a background risk of 3% or more for a serious birth defect, even when mom doesn't take a drug of any kind. If you are pregnant or planning a pregnancy, always let your healthcare provider know before taking any drug, prescription or non-prescription, or herbal remedy.

CVS® Sinus Congestion & Pain Caplets Daytime & Nighttime

Active Ingredient:	Pregnancy Risk Category:
Daytime:	
Acetaminophen	B
Phenylephrine Hcl	C
Nighttime:	
Acetaminophen	B
Phenylephrine Hcl	C
Chlorpheniramine maleate	B

Helpful Hints and Reminders: Each pregnancy risk category (**A**, **B**, **C**, **D**, or **X**) is explained on the last page of this section.

Remember: All pregnancies have a background risk of 3% or more for a serious birth defect, even when mom doesn't take a drug of any kind. If you are pregnant or planning a pregnancy, always let your healthcare provider know before taking any drug, prescription or non-prescription, or herbal remedy.

DayQuil® Sinus LiquiCaps

Active Ingredient:	Pregnancy Risk Category:
Acetaminophen	B
Phenylephrine Hcl	C

Helpful Hints and Reminders: Each pregnancy risk category (**A**, **B**, **C**, **D**, or **X**) is explained on the last page of this section.

Remember: All pregnancies have a background risk of 3% or more for a serious birth defect, even when mom doesn't take a drug of any kind. If you are pregnant or planning a pregnancy, always let your healthcare provider know before taking any drug, prescription or non-prescription, or herbal remedy.

Dimetapp® Cold & Allergy Chewable Tablets

Active Ingredient:	Pregnancy Risk Category:
Brompheniramine maleate	C
Phenylephrine Hcl	C

Helpful Hints and Reminders: Each pregnancy risk category (**A**, **B**, **C**, **D**, or **X**) is explained on the last page of this section.

Remember: All pregnancies have a background risk of 3% or more for a serious birth defect, even when mom doesn't take a drug of any kind. If you are pregnant or planning a pregnancy, always let your healthcare provider know before taking any drug, prescription or non-prescription, or herbal remedy.

Dimetapp® Cold & Allergy Liquid

Active Ingredient:	Pregnancy Risk Category:
Brompheniramine maleate	C
Phenylephrine Hcl	C

Helpful Hints and Reminders: Each pregnancy risk category (**A**, **B**, **C**, **D**, or **X**) is explained on the last page of this section.

Remember: All pregnancies have a background risk of 3% or more for a serious birth defect, even when mom doesn't take a drug of any kind. If you are pregnant or planning a pregnancy, always let your healthcare provider know before taking any drug, prescription or non-prescription, or herbal remedy.

Dimetapp® Cold & Cough

Active Ingredient:	Pregnancy Risk Category:
Brompheniramine maleate	C
Phenylephrine Hcl	C
Dextromethorphan	C

Helpful Hints and Reminders: Each pregnancy risk category (**A**, **B**, **C**, **D**, or **X**) is explained on the last page of this section.

Remember: All pregnancies have a background risk of 3% or more for a serious birth defect, even when mom doesn't take a drug of any kind. If you are pregnant or planning a pregnancy, always let your healthcare provider know before taking any drug, prescription or non-prescription, or herbal remedy.

Dimetapp® Long Acting Cough Plus Cold

Active Ingredient:	Pregnancy Risk Category:
Dextromethorphan	C
Chlorpheniramine	B

Helpful Hints and Reminders: Each pregnancy risk category (**A**, **B**, **C**, **D**, or **X**) is explained on the last page of this section.

Remember: All pregnancies have a background risk of 3% or more for a serious birth defect, even when mom doesn't take a drug of any kind. If you are pregnant or planning a pregnancy, always let your healthcare provider know before taking any drug, prescription or non-prescription, or herbal remedy.

Dimetapp® Nighttime Cold & Congestion

Active Ingredient:	Pregnancy Risk Category:
Phenylephrine Hcl	C
Diphenhydramine Hcl	B

Helpful Hints and Reminders: Each pregnancy risk category (**A**, **B**, **C**, **D**, or **X**) is explained on the last page of this section.

Remember: All pregnancies have a background risk of 3% or more for a serious birth defect, even when mom doesn't take a drug of any kind. If you are pregnant or planning a pregnancy, always let your healthcare provider know before taking any drug, prescription or non-prescription, or herbal remedy.

Dristan® Cold Multi-Symptom Nasal Decongestant Coated Tablets

Active Ingredient:	Pregnancy Risk Category:
Acetaminophen	B
Phenylephrine Hcl	C
Chlorpheniramine maleate	B

Helpful Hints and Reminders: Each pregnancy risk category (**A**, **B**, **C**, **D**, or **X**) is explained on the last page of this section.

Remember: All pregnancies have a background risk of 3% or more for a serious birth defect, even when mom doesn't take a drug of any kind. If you are pregnant or planning a pregnancy, always let your healthcare provider know before taking any drug, prescription or non-prescription, or herbal remedy.

Equate® 24 Hour Non-Drowsy Allergy Relief, Loratadine Tablets 10 Mg

Active Ingredient:	Pregnancy Risk Category:
Loratadine	B

Helpful Hints and Reminders: Each pregnancy risk category (**A**, **B**, **C**, **D**, or **X**) is explained on the last page of this section.

Remember: All pregnancies have a background risk of 3% or more for a serious birth defect, even when mom doesn't take a drug of any kind. If you are pregnant or planning a pregnancy, always let your healthcare provider know before taking any drug, prescription or non-prescription, or herbal remedy.

Equate® Allergy & Sinus Medication Tablets

Active Ingredient:	Pregnancy Risk Category:
Diphenhydramine Hcl	B
Phenylephrine Hcl	C

Helpful Hints and Reminders: Each pregnancy risk category (**A**, **B**, **C**, **D**, or **X**) is explained on the last page of this section.

Remember: All pregnancies have a background risk of 3% or more for a serious birth defect, even when mom doesn't take a drug of any kind. If you are pregnant or planning a pregnancy, always let your healthcare provider know before taking any drug, prescription or non-prescription, or herbal remedy.

Equate® Allergy 24 Hour Indoor & Outdoor Tablets

Active Ingredient:	Pregnancy Risk Category:
Cetirizine Hcl	B

Helpful Hints and Reminders: Each pregnancy risk category (**A**, **B**, **C**, **D**, or **X**) is explained on the last page of this section.

Remember: All pregnancies have a background risk of 3% or more for a serious birth defect, even when mom doesn't take a drug of any kind. If you are pregnant or planning a pregnancy, always let your healthcare provider know before taking any drug, prescription or non-prescription, or herbal remedy.

Equate® Allergy Medication 25 Mg Antihistamine Capsules

Active Ingredient:	Pregnancy Risk Category:
Diphenhydramine Hcl	B

Helpful Hints and Reminders: Each pregnancy risk category (**A**, **B**, **C**, **D**, or **X**) is explained on the last page of this section.

Remember: All pregnancies have a background risk of 3% or more for a serious birth defect, even when mom doesn't take a drug of any kind. If you are pregnant or planning a pregnancy, always let your healthcare provider know before taking any drug, prescription or non-prescription, or herbal remedy.

Equate® Allergy Relief Liquid

Active Ingredient:	Pregnancy Risk Category:
Cetirizine Hcl	B

Helpful Hints and Reminders: Each pregnancy risk category (**A**, **B**, **C**, **D**, or **X**) is explained on the last page of this section.

Remember: All pregnancies have a background risk of 3% or more for a serious birth defect, even when mom doesn't take a drug of any kind. If you are pregnant or planning a pregnancy, always let your healthcare provider know before taking any drug, prescription or non-prescription, or herbal remedy.

Equate® Allergy/Sinus Headache Pain Reliever Caplets

Active Ingredient:	Pregnancy Risk Category:
Diphenhydramine Hcl	B
Acetaminophen	B
Phenylephrine Hcl	C

Helpful Hints and Reminders: Each pregnancy risk category (**A**, **B**, **C**, **D**, or **X**) is explained on the last page of this section.

Remember: All pregnancies have a background risk of 3% or more for a serious birth defect, even when mom doesn't take a drug of any kind. If you are pregnant or planning a pregnancy, always let your healthcare provider know before taking any drug, prescription or non-prescription, or herbal remedy.

Equate® Allergy-D Original Antihistamine/ Nasal Decongestant 12 Hour Tablets

Active Ingredient:	Pregnancy Risk Category:
Cetirizine Hcl	B
Pseudoephedrine Hcl	C

Helpful Hints and Reminders: Each pregnancy risk category (**A**, **B**, **C**, **D**, or **X**) is explained on the last page of this section.

Remember: All pregnancies have a background risk of 3% or more for a serious birth defect, even when mom doesn't take a drug of any kind. If you are pregnant or planning a pregnancy, always let your healthcare provider know before taking any drug, prescription or non-prescription, or herbal remedy.

Equate® Antihistabs Cold & Allergy Relief Tablets

Active Ingredient:	Pregnancy Risk Category:
Chlorpheniramine maleate	B
Phenylephrine Hcl	C

Helpful Hints and Reminders: Each pregnancy risk category (**A**, **B**, **C**, **D**, or **X**) is explained on the last page of this section.

Remember: All pregnancies have a background risk of 3% or more for a serious birth defect, even when mom doesn't take a drug of any kind. If you are pregnant or planning a pregnancy, always let your healthcare provider know before taking any drug, prescription or non-prescription, or herbal remedy.

Equate® Severe Allergy & Sinus Headache Maximum Strength Caplets

Active Ingredient:	Pregnancy Risk Category:
Acetaminophen	B
Diphenhydramine Hcl	B
Phenylephrine Hcl	C

Helpful Hints and Reminders: Each pregnancy risk category (**A**, **B**, **C**, **D**, or **X**) is explained on the last page of this section.

Remember: All pregnancies have a background risk of 3% or more for a serious birth defect, even when mom doesn't take a drug of any kind. If you are pregnant or planning a pregnancy, always let your healthcare provider know before taking any drug, prescription or non-prescription, or herbal remedy.

Equate® Suphedrine PE Sinus & Allergy Tablets Antihistamine/Nasal Decongestant

Active Ingredient:	Pregnancy Risk Category:
Chlorpheniramine maleate	B
Phenylephrine Hcl	C

Helpful Hints and Reminders: Each pregnancy risk category (**A**, **B**, **C**, **D**, or **X**) is explained on the last page of this section.

Remember: All pregnancies have a background risk of 3% or more for a serious birth defect, even when mom doesn't take a drug of any kind. If you are pregnant or planning a pregnancy, always let your healthcare provider know before taking any drug, prescription or non-prescription, or herbal remedy.

Equate® Tutti Frutti Flavor Allergy Relief Chewable Tablets

Active Ingredient:	Pregnancy Risk Category:
Cetirizine Hcl	B

Kirkland Signature™ Allerclear® Non-Drowsy **19**

Helpful Hints and Reminders: Each pregnancy risk category (**A**, **B**, **C**, **D**, or **X**) is explained on the last page of this section.

Remember: All pregnancies have a background risk of 3% or more for a serious birth defect, even when mom doesn't take a drug of any kind. If you are pregnant or planning a pregnancy, always let your healthcare provider know before taking any drug, prescription or non-prescription, or herbal remedy.

Excedrin® Sinus Headache Caplets & Tablets

Active Ingredient:	Pregnancy Risk Category:
Acetaminophen	B
Phenylephrine	C

Helpful Hints and Reminders: Each pregnancy risk category (**A**, **B**, **C**, **D**, or **X**) is explained on the last page of this section.

Remember: All pregnancies have a background risk of 3% or more for a serious birth defect, even when mom doesn't take a drug of any kind. If you are pregnant or planning a pregnancy, always let your healthcare provider know before taking any drug, prescription or non-prescription, or herbal remedy.

Kirkland Signature™ AllerClear® Non-Drowsy

Active Ingredient:	Pregnancy Risk Category:
Loratadine	B

Helpful Hints and Reminders: Each pregnancy risk category (**A**, **B**, **C**, **D**, or **X**) is explained on the last page of this section.

Remember: All pregnancies have a background risk of 3% or more for a serious birth defect, even when mom doesn't take a drug of any kind. If you are pregnant or planning a pregnancy, always let your healthcare provider know before taking any drug, prescription or non-prescription, or herbal remedy.

Kirkland Signature™ Allergy Medicine Antihistamine 25 Mg Allergy Relief

Active Ingredient:	Pregnancy Risk Category:
Diphenhydramine Hcl	B

Helpful Hints and Reminders: Each pregnancy risk category (**A**, **B**, **C**, **D**, or **X**) is explained on the last page of this section.

Remember: All pregnancies have a background risk of 3% or more for a serious birth defect, even when mom doesn't take a drug of any kind. If you are pregnant or planning a pregnancy, always let your healthcare provider know before taking any drug, prescription or non-prescription, or herbal remedy.

Kirkland Signature™ Aller-Tec™ Cetirizine HCL Antihistamine

Active Ingredient:	Pregnancy Risk Category:
Cetirizine Hcl	B

Helpful Hints and Reminders: Each pregnancy risk category (**A**, **B**, **C**, **D**, or **X**) is explained on the last page of this section.

Remember: All pregnancies have a background risk of 3% or more for a serious birth defect, even when mom doesn't take a drug of any kind. If you are pregnant or planning a pregnancy, always let your healthcare provider know before taking any drug, prescription or non-prescription, or herbal remedy.

Kirkland Signature™ Suphedrine PE, Nasal & Sinus Decongestant Formula

Active Ingredient:	Pregnancy Risk Category:
Phenylephrine Hcl	C

Helpful Hints and Reminders: Each pregnancy risk category (**A**, **B**, **C**, **D**, or **X**) is explained on the last page of this section.

Remember: All pregnancies have a background risk of 3% or more for a serious birth defect, even when mom doesn't take a drug of any kind. If you are pregnant or planning a pregnancy, always let your healthcare provider know before taking any drug, prescription or non-prescription, or herbal remedy.

NasalCrom® Nasal Allergy Symptom Controller Spray

Active Ingredient:	Pregnancy Risk Category:
Cromolyn sodium	B

Helpful Hints and Reminders: Each pregnancy risk category (**A**, **B**, **C**, **D**, or **X**) is explained on the last page of this section.

Remember: All pregnancies have a background risk of 3% or more for a serious birth defect, even when mom doesn't take a drug of any kind. If you are pregnant or planning a pregnancy, always let your healthcare provider know before taking any drug, prescription or non-prescription, or herbal remedy.

NyQuil® Sinus LiquiCaps

Active Ingredient:	Pregnancy Risk Category:
Acetaminophen	B
Doxylamine succinate	A
Phenylephrine Hcl	C

Helpful Hints and Reminders: Each pregnancy risk category (**A**, **B**, **C**, **D**, or **X**) is explained on the last page of this section.

Remember: All pregnancies have a background risk of 3% or more for a serious birth defect, even when mom doesn't take a drug of any kind. If you are pregnant or planning a pregnancy, always let your healthcare provider know before taking any drug, prescription or non-prescription, or herbal remedy.

Primatene® Mist

Active Ingredient:	Pregnancy Risk Category:
Epinephrine	C

Helpful Hints and Reminders: Each pregnancy risk category (**A**, **B**, **C**, **D**, or **X**) is explained on the last page of this section.

Remember: All pregnancies have a background risk of 3% or more for a serious birth defect, even when mom doesn't take a drug of any kind. If you are pregnant or planning a pregnancy, always let your healthcare provider know before taking any drug, prescription or non-prescription, or herbal remedy.

Rite Aid® Mucus Relief Sinus Expectorant/Decongestant

Active Ingredient:	Pregnancy Risk Category:
Guaifenesin	C
Phenylephrine Hcl	C

Helpful Hints and Reminders: Each pregnancy risk category (**A**, **B**, **C**, **D**, or **X**) is explained on the last page of this section.

Remember: All pregnancies have a background risk of 3% or more for a serious birth defect, even when mom doesn't take a drug of any kind. If you are pregnant or planning a pregnancy, always let your healthcare provider know before taking any drug, prescription or non-prescription, or herbal remedy.

Rite Aid® Nose Drops

Active Ingredient:	Pregnancy Risk Category:
Phenylephrine Hcl	C

Helpful Hints and Reminders: Each pregnancy risk category (**A**, **B**, **C**, **D**, or **X**) is explained on the last page of this section.

Remember: All pregnancies have a background risk of 3% or more for a serious birth defect, even when mom doesn't take a drug of any kind. If you are pregnant or planning a pregnancy, always let your healthcare provider know before taking any drug, prescription or non-prescription, or herbal remedy.

Robitussin® Cough & Allergy

Active Ingredient:	Pregnancy Risk Category:
Chlorpheniramine maleate	B
Dextromethorphan Hbr	C
Phenylephrine Hcl	C

Helpful Hints and Reminders: Each pregnancy risk category (**A**, **B**, **C**, **D**, or **X**) is explained on the last page of this section.

Remember: All pregnancies have a background risk of 3% or more for a serious birth defect, even when mom doesn't take a drug of any kind. If you are pregnant or planning a pregnancy, always let your healthcare provider know before taking any drug, prescription or non-prescription, or herbal remedy.

Robitussin® Cough & Cold Long Acting

Active Ingredient:	Pregnancy Risk Category:
Dextromethorphan Hbr	C
Chlorpheniramine maleate	B

Helpful Hints and Reminders: Each pregnancy risk category (**A**, **B**, **C**, **D**, or **X**) is explained on the last page of this section.

Remember: All pregnancies have a background risk of 3% or more for a serious birth defect, even when mom doesn't take a drug of any kind. If you are pregnant or planning a pregnancy, always let your healthcare provider know before taking any drug, prescription or non-prescription, or herbal remedy.

Robitussin® Nighttime Cough & Cold

Active Ingredient:	Pregnancy Risk Category:
Phenylephrine Hcl	C
Diphenhydramine Hcl	B

Helpful Hints and Reminders: Each pregnancy risk category (**A**, **B**, **C**, **D**, or **X**) is explained on the last page of this section.

Remember: All pregnancies have a background risk of 3% or more for a serious birth defect, even when mom doesn't take a drug of any kind. If you are pregnant or planning a pregnancy, always let your healthcare provider know before taking any drug, prescription or non-prescription, or herbal remedy.

Sudafed PE® Maximum Strength Sinus & Allergy Tablets

Active Ingredient:	Pregnancy Risk Category:
Chlorpheniramine maleate	B
Phenylephrine Hcl	C

Helpful Hints and Reminders: Each pregnancy risk category (**A**, **B**, **C**, **D**, or **X**) is explained on the last page of this section.

Remember: All pregnancies have a background risk of 3% or more for a serious birth defect, even when mom doesn't take a drug of any kind. If you are pregnant or planning a pregnancy, always let your healthcare provider know before taking any drug, prescription or non-prescription, or herbal remedy.

Sudafed PE® Nasal Decongestant Tablets

Active Ingredient:	Pregnancy Risk Category:
Phenylephrine Hcl	C

Helpful Hints and Reminders: Each pregnancy risk category (**A**, **B**, **C**, **D**, or **X**) is explained on the last page of this section.

Remember: All pregnancies have a background risk of 3% or more for a serious birth defect, even when mom doesn't take a drug of any kind. If you are pregnant or planning a pregnancy, always let your healthcare provider know before taking any drug, prescription or non-prescription, or herbal remedy.

Sudafed PE® Non-Drying Sinus Caplets

Active Ingredient:	Pregnancy Risk Category:
Phenylephrine Hcl	C
Guaifenesin	C

Helpful Hints and Reminders: Each pregnancy risk category (**A**, **B**, **C**, **D**, or **X**) is explained on the last page of this section.

Remember: All pregnancies have a background risk of 3% or more for a serious birth defect, even when mom doesn't take a drug of any kind. If you are pregnant or planning a pregnancy, always let your healthcare provider know before taking any drug, prescription or non-prescription, or herbal remedy.

Sudafed PE® Sinus Headache Caplets

Active Ingredient:	Pregnancy Risk Category:
Acetaminophen	B
Phenylephrine Hcl	C

Helpful Hints and Reminders: Each pregnancy risk category (**A**, **B**, **C**, **D**, or **X**) is explained on the last page of this section.

Remember: All pregnancies have a background risk of 3% or more for a serious birth defect, even when mom doesn't take a drug of any kind. If you are pregnant or planning a pregnancy, always let your healthcare provider know before taking any drug, prescription or non-prescription, or herbal remedy.

Sudafed PE® Triple Action™ Caplets

Active Ingredient:	Pregnancy Risk Category:
Acetaminophen	B
Guaifenesin	C
Phenylephrine Hcl	C

Helpful Hints and Reminders: Each pregnancy risk category (**A**, **B**, **C**, **D**, or **X**) is explained on the last page of this section.

Remember: All pregnancies have a background risk of 3% or more for a serious birth defect, even when mom doesn't take a drug of any kind. If you are pregnant or planning a pregnancy, always let your healthcare provider know before taking any drug, prescription or non-prescription, or herbal remedy.

Sudafed® 12 Hour Tablets

Active Ingredient:	Pregnancy Risk Category:
Pseudoephedrine Hcl	C

Helpful Hints and Reminders: Each pregnancy risk category (**A**, **B**, **C**, **D**, or **X**) is explained on the last page of this section.

Remember: All pregnancies have a background risk of 3% or more for a serious birth defect, even when mom doesn't take a drug of any kind. If you are pregnant or planning a pregnancy, always let your healthcare provider know before taking any drug, prescription or non-prescription, or herbal remedy.

Sudafed® 24 Hour Tablets

Active Ingredient:	Pregnancy Risk Category:
Pseudoephedrine Hcl	C

Helpful Hints and Reminders: Each pregnancy risk category (**A**, **B**, **C**, **D**, or **X**) is explained on the last page of this section.

Remember: All pregnancies have a background risk of 3% or more for a serious birth defect, even when mom doesn't take a drug of any kind.

If you are pregnant or planning a pregnancy, always let your healthcare provider know before taking any drug, prescription or non-prescription, or herbal remedy.

Sudafed® Nasal Decongestant Tablets

Active Ingredient:	Pregnancy Risk Category:
Pseudoephedrine Hcl	C

Helpful Hints and Reminders: Each pregnancy risk category (**A**, **B**, **C**, **D**, or **X**) is explained on the last page of this section.

Remember: All pregnancies have a background risk of 3% or more for a serious birth defect, even when mom doesn't take a drug of any kind. If you are pregnant or planning a pregnancy, always let your healthcare provider know before taking any drug, prescription or non-prescription, or herbal remedy.

Sudafed® Sinus Pain 12 Hour Caplet

Active Ingredient:	Pregnancy Risk Category:
Pseudoephedrine Hcl	C
Naproxen sodium	Naproxen sodium has two pregnancy risk categories: **C** when used in the first or second trimesters of pregnancy; **D** if used in the third trimester. (See Helpful Hints below.)

Helpful Hints and Reminders: Each pregnancy risk category (**A**, **B**, **C**, **D**, or **X**) is explained on the last page of this section.

1. Naproxen sodium is a member of the non-steroidal, anti-inflammatory family of drugs, or NSAIDs. Members of this family of drugs should not be used during the third trimester of pregnancy (last 12 weeks) unless specifically prescribed by a clinician. See the Appendix for "Non-Steroidal, Anti-Inflammatory Drugs (NSAIDs) in Pregnancy," which describes the serious problems these drugs may cause for unborn babies when taken in the third trimester of pregnancy.

2. Women attempting to conceive should not use any NSAID, including Naproxen sodium, because of the findings in animals that these drugs may block implantation of the early embryo in the wall of the uterus, in effect preventing pregnancy.

Remember: All pregnancies have a background risk of 3% or more for a serious birth defect, even when mom doesn't take a drug of any kind. If you are pregnant or planning a pregnancy, always let your healthcare provider know before taking any drug, prescription or non-prescription, or herbal remedy.

Sudafed® Triple Action™ Caplets

Active Ingredient:	Pregnancy Risk Category:
Acetaminophen	B
Guaifenesin	C
Pseudoephedrine Hcl	C

Helpful Hints and Reminders: Each pregnancy risk category (**A**, **B**, **C**, **D**, or **X**) is explained on the last page of this section.

Remember: All pregnancies have a background risk of 3% or more for a serious birth defect, even when mom doesn't take a drug of any kind. If you are pregnant or planning a pregnancy, always let your healthcare provider know before taking any drug, prescription or non-prescription, or herbal remedy.

Target® Allergy Relief Capsules

Active Ingredient:	Pregnancy Risk Category:
Diphenhydramine Hcl	B

Helpful Hints and Reminders: Each pregnancy risk category (**A**, **B**, **C**, **D**, or **X**) is explained on the last page of this section.

Remember: All pregnancies have a background risk of 3% or more for a serious birth defect, even when mom doesn't take a drug of any kind. If you are pregnant or planning a pregnancy, always let your healthcare provider know before taking any drug, prescription or non-prescription, or herbal remedy.

Tavist® Allergy Tablets

Target® Maximum Strength Nasal Decongestant PE Tablets

Active Ingredient:	Pregnancy Risk Category:
Phenylephrine Hcl	C

Helpful Hints and Reminders: Each pregnancy risk category (**A**, **B**, **C**, **D**, or **X**) is explained on the last page of this section.

Remember: All pregnancies have a background risk of 3% or more for a serious birth defect, even when mom doesn't take a drug of any kind. If you are pregnant or planning a pregnancy, always let your healthcare provider know before taking any drug, prescription or non-prescription, or herbal remedy.

Target® Sinus Congestion & Pain Cool Ice® Caplets

Active Ingredient:	Pregnancy Risk Category:
Acetaminophen	B
Phenylephrine Hcl	C

Helpful Hints and Reminders: Each pregnancy risk category (**A**, **B**, **C**, **D**, or **X**) is explained on the last page of this section.

Remember: All pregnancies have a background risk of 3% or more for a serious birth defect, even when mom doesn't take a drug of any kind. If you are pregnant or planning a pregnancy, always let your healthcare provider know before taking any drug, prescription or non-prescription, or herbal remedy.

Tavist® Allergy Tablets

Active Ingredient:	Pregnancy Risk Category:
Clemastine	B

Helpful Hints and Reminders: Each pregnancy risk category (**A**, **B**, **C**, **D**, or **X**) is explained on the last page of this section.

Remember: All pregnancies have a background risk of 3% or more for a serious birth defect, even when mom doesn't take a drug of any kind. If you are pregnant or planning a pregnancy, always let your healthcare provider know before taking any drug, prescription or non-prescription, or herbal remedy.

Theraflu® Cold & Sore Throat

Active Ingredient:	Pregnancy Risk Category:
Acetaminophen	B
Pheniramine maleate	C
Phenylephrine Hcl	C

Helpful Hints and Reminders: Each pregnancy risk category (**A**, **B**, **C**, **D**, or **X**) is explained on the last page of this section.

Remember: All pregnancies have a background risk of 3% or more for a serious birth defect, even when mom doesn't take a drug of any kind. If you are pregnant or planning a pregnancy, always let your healthcare provider know before taking any drug, prescription or non-prescription, or herbal remedy.

Tylenol® Allergy Multi-Symptom

Active Ingredient:	Pregnancy Risk Category:
Acetaminophen	B
Phenylephrine Hcl	C
Chlorpheniramine maleate	B

Helpful Hints and Reminders: Each pregnancy risk category (**A**, **B**, **C**, **D**, or **X**) is explained on the last page of this section.

Remember: All pregnancies have a background risk of 3% or more for a serious birth defect, even when mom doesn't take a drug of any kind. If you are pregnant or planning a pregnancy, always let your healthcare provider know before taking any drug, prescription or non-prescription, or herbal remedy.

Tylenol® Sinus Congestion and Pain Day/Night Pack　　**31**

Tylenol® Allergy Multi-Symptom Nighttime

Active Ingredient:	Pregnancy Risk Category:
Acetaminophen	B
Diphenhydramine Hcl	B
Phenylephrine Hcl	C

Helpful Hints and Reminders: Each pregnancy risk category (**A**, **B**, **C**, **D**, or **X**) is explained on the last page of this section.

Remember: All pregnancies have a background risk of 3% or more for a serious birth defect, even when mom doesn't take a drug of any kind. If you are pregnant or planning a pregnancy, always let your healthcare provider know before taking any drug, prescription or non-prescription, or herbal remedy.

Tylenol® Sinus Congestion and Pain Day/Night Pack

Active Ingredient:	Pregnancy Risk Category:
Daytime:	
Acetaminophen	B
Phenylephrine Hcl	C
Nighttime:	
Acetaminophen	B
Phenylephrine Hcl	C
Chlorpheniramine maleate	B

Helpful Hints and Reminders: Each pregnancy risk category (**A**, **B**, **C**, **D**, or **X**) is explained on the last page of this section.

Remember: All pregnancies have a background risk of 3% or more for a serious birth defect, even when mom doesn't take a drug of any kind. If you are pregnant or planning a pregnancy, always let your healthcare provider know before taking any drug, prescription or non-prescription, or herbal remedy.

Tylenol® Sinus Congestion and Pain Daytime

Active Ingredient:	Pregnancy Risk Category:
Acetaminophen	B
Phenylephrine Hcl	C

Helpful Hints and Reminders: Each pregnancy risk category (**A**, **B**, **C**, **D**, or **X**) is explained on the last page of this section.

Remember: All pregnancies have a background risk of 3% or more for a serious birth defect, even when mom doesn't take a drug of any kind. If you are pregnant or planning a pregnancy, always let your healthcare provider know before taking any drug, prescription or non-prescription, or herbal remedy.

Tylenol® Sinus Congestion and Pain Nighttime

Active Ingredient:	Pregnancy Risk Category:
Acetaminophen	B
Phenylephrine Hcl	C
Chlorpheniramine maleate	B

Helpful Hints and Reminders: Each pregnancy risk category (**A**, **B**, **C**, **D**, or **X**) is explained on the last page of this section.

Remember: All pregnancies have a background risk of 3% or more for a serious birth defect, even when mom doesn't take a drug of any kind. If you are pregnant or planning a pregnancy, always let your healthcare provider know before taking any drug, prescription or non-prescription, or herbal remedy.

Tylenol® Sinus Congestion and Pain Severe

Active Ingredient:	Pregnancy Risk Category:
Acetaminophen	B
Phenylephrine Hcl	C
Guaifenesin	C

Walgreens® WAL-ITIN® Indoor and Outdoor Allergy 24 Hour Relief 33

Helpful Hints and Reminders: Each pregnancy risk category (**A**, **B**, **C**, **D**, or **X**) is explained on the last page of this section.

Remember: All pregnancies have a background risk of 3% or more for a serious birth defect, even when mom doesn't take a drug of any kind. If you are pregnant or planning a pregnancy, always let your healthcare provider know before taking any drug, prescription or non-prescription, or herbal remedy.

Up & Up™ Allergy & Cold Relief

Active Ingredient:	Pregnancy Risk Category:
Acetaminophen	B
Diphenhydramine Hcl	B
Phenylephrine Hcl	C

Helpful Hints and Reminders: Each pregnancy risk category (**A**, **B**, **C**, **D**, or **X**) is explained on the last page of this section.

Remember: All pregnancies have a background risk of 3% or more for a serious birth defect, even when mom doesn't take a drug of any kind. If you are pregnant or planning a pregnancy, always let your healthcare provider know before taking any drug, prescription or non-prescription, or herbal remedy.

Walgreens® WAL-ITIN® Indoor and Outdoor Allergy 24 Hour Relief

Active Ingredient:	Pregnancy Risk Category:
Loratadine	B

Helpful Hints and Reminders: Each pregnancy risk category (**A**, **B**, **C**, **D**, or **X**) is explained on the last page of this section.

Remember: All pregnancies have a background risk of 3% or more for a serious birth defect, even when mom doesn't take a drug of any kind. If you are pregnant or planning a pregnancy, always let your healthcare provider know before taking any drug, prescription or non-prescription, or herbal remedy.

Walgreens® Wal-Zyr™ All Day Allergy Tablets

Active Ingredient:	Pregnancy Risk Category:
Cetirizine Hcl	B

Helpful Hints and Reminders: Each pregnancy risk category (**A**, **B**, **C**, **D**, or **X**) is explained on the last page of this section.

Remember: All pregnancies have a background risk of 3% or more for a serious birth defect, even when mom doesn't take a drug of any kind. If you are pregnant or planning a pregnancy, always let your healthcare provider know before taking any drug, prescription or non-prescription, or herbal remedy.

XL-3® Cold Medicine Tablets

Active Ingredient:	Pregnancy Risk Category:
Acetaminophen	B
Chlorpheniramine maleate	B
Phenylephrine Hcl	C

Helpful Hints and Reminders: Each pregnancy risk category (**A**, **B**, **C**, **D**, or **X**) is explained on the last page of this section.

Remember: All pregnancies have a background risk of 3% or more for a serious birth defect, even when mom doesn't take a drug of any kind. If you are pregnant or planning a pregnancy, always let your healthcare provider know before taking any drug, prescription or non-prescription, or herbal remedy.

Zyrtec® 10 Mg Liquid Gels

Active Ingredient:	Pregnancy Risk Category:
Cetirizine Hcl	B

Helpful Hints and Reminders: Each pregnancy risk category (**A**, **B**, **C**, **D**, or **X**) is explained on the last page of this section.

Remember: All pregnancies have a background risk of 3% or more for a serious birth defect, even when mom doesn't take a drug of any kind.

Zyrtec-D®

If you are pregnant or planning a pregnancy, always let your healthcare provider know before taking any drug, prescription or non-prescription, or herbal remedy.

Zyrtec® Itchy Eye Drops

Active Ingredient:	Pregnancy Risk Category:
Ketotifen	C

Helpful Hints and Reminders: Each pregnancy risk category (**A**, **B**, **C**, **D**, or **X**) is explained on the last page of this section.

Remember: All pregnancies have a background risk of 3% or more for a serious birth defect, even when mom doesn't take a drug of any kind. If you are pregnant or planning a pregnancy, always let your healthcare provider know before taking any drug, prescription or non-prescription, or herbal remedy.

Zyrtec® Tablets

Active Ingredient:	Pregnancy Risk Category:
Cetirizine Hcl	B

Helpful Hints and Reminders: Each pregnancy risk category (**A**, **B**, **C**, **D**, or **X**) is explained on the last page of this section.

Remember: All pregnancies have a background risk of 3% or more for a serious birth defect, even when mom doesn't take a drug of any kind. If you are pregnant or planning a pregnancy, always let your healthcare provider know before taking any drug, prescription or non-prescription, or herbal remedy.

Zyrtec-D®

Active Ingredient:	Pregnancy Risk Category:
Cetirizine Hcl	B
Pseudoephedrine Hcl	C

Helpful Hints and Reminders: Each pregnancy risk category (**A**, **B**, **C**, **D**, or **X**) is explained on the last page of this section.

Remember: All pregnancies have a background risk of 3% or more for a serious birth defect, even when mom doesn't take a drug of any kind. If you are pregnant or planning a pregnancy, always let your healthcare provider know before taking any drug, prescription or non-prescription, or herbal remedy.

The FDA's Pregnancy Risk Categories: A, B, C, D, X

Adapted to the Active Ingredients in Nonprescription drugs

Category A: Controlled studies using the active ingredient in pregnant women have not shown harmful fetal effects throughout pregnancy, and the possibility of fetal harm seems remote. My comment: *Though apparently safe, these active ingredients should still only be used in pregnancy when clearly indicated.*

Category B: Either studies have shown no evidence of fetal harm when using the active ingredient in pregnant animals, but no controlled studies have been done in pregnant women, **or** studies have shown evidence of fetal harm when using the active ingredient in pregnant animals, but controlled studies in pregnant women have not shown evidence of fetal harm. My comment: *These active ingredients should only be used in pregnancy when clearly indicated.*

Category C: Either studies have shown evidence of fetal harm when using the active ingredient in pregnant animals, but no controlled studies have been done in pregnant women, **or** studies using the active ingredient in pregnant animals have not been done, and studies of pregnant women are insufficient to reach a conclusion. These active ingredients should only be used by a pregnant woman if the potential benefit justifies the potential risk of fetal harm, which, in many cases, is unknown. My comment: *It's impossible to calculate the potential risk of fetal harm when, in many cases, it's unknown. Thus, these active ingredients should only be used in pregnancy when clearly needed.*

Category D: Studies have shown evidence of fetal harm when using the active ingredient in pregnant women. However, the potential benefit of using the active ingredient in some life-threatening situations for

mom may outweigh the potential risk of fetal harm. For example, when mom requires cancer treatment or when she has a serious disease for which safer active ingredients cannot be used or are less effective. My comment: *These exceptional indications rarely occur when considering a nonprescription drug in pregnancy.*

Category X: My comment: *Because the risk of fetal harm is too high, no Category X active ingredients have been approved for use in nonprescription drugs.*

Active Ingredients Assigned Two Pregnancy Risk Categories: Some active ingredients have two pregnancy risk categories, depending on which trimester of pregnancy the active ingredient is used. For example, naproxen sodium, the active ingredient in Aleve, belongs to Category **B** when used in the first and second trimesters of pregnancy. If used in the third trimester, however, the active ingredient belongs to Category **D**. My comment: *This means naproxen sodium should not be used in the third trimester unless prescribed by a physician who has advised his or her patient of the risks involved.*

Section 2: Cough, Cold & Flu

4-Way® Fast Acting Nasal Spray: Nasal Decongestant

Active Ingredient:	Pregnancy Risk Category:
Phenylephrine Hcl	C

Helpful Hints and Reminders: Each pregnancy risk category (**A**, **B**, **C**, **D**, or **X**) is explained on the last page of this section.

Remember: All pregnancies have a background risk of 3% or more for a serious birth defect, even when mom doesn't take a drug of any kind. If you are pregnant or planning a pregnancy, always let your healthcare provider know before taking any drug, prescription or non-prescription, or herbal remedy.

4-Way® Menthol: Nasal Decongestant

Active Ingredient:	Pregnancy Risk Category:
Phenylephrine Hcl	C

Helpful Hints and Reminders: Each pregnancy risk category (**A**, **B**, **C**, **D**, or **X**) is explained on the last page of this section.

Remember: All pregnancies have a background risk of 3% or more for a serious birth defect, even when mom doesn't take a drug of any kind.

If you are pregnant or planning a pregnancy, always let your healthcare provider know before taking any drug, prescription or non-prescription, or herbal remedy.

4-Way® Moisturizing Relief Nasal Decongestant

Active Ingredient:	Pregnancy Risk Category:
Xylometazoline Hcl	C

Helpful Hints and Reminders: Each pregnancy risk category (**A**, **B**, **C**, **D**, or **X**) is explained on the last page of this section.

Remember: All pregnancies have a background risk of 3% or more for a serious birth defect, even when mom doesn't take a drug of any kind. If you are pregnant or planning a pregnancy, always let your healthcare provider know before taking any drug, prescription or non-prescription, or herbal remedy.

Actifed® Cold & Allergy Tablets

Active Ingredient:	Pregnancy Risk Category:
Chlorpheniramine maleate	B
Phenylephrine Hcl	C

Helpful Hints and Reminders: Each pregnancy risk category (**A**, **B**, **C**, **D**, or **X**) is explained on the last page of this section.

Remember: All pregnancies have a background risk of 3% or more for a serious birth defect, even when mom doesn't take a drug of any kind. If you are pregnant or planning a pregnancy, always let your healthcare provider know before taking any drug, prescription or non-prescription, or herbal remedy.

Advil® Cold & Sinus Caplets & Liqui-Gels®

Active Ingredient:	Pregnancy Risk Category:
Pseudoephedrine Hcl	C
Ibuprofen	Ibuprofen has two pregnancy risk categories: **B** when used in the first or second trimesters of pregnancy; **D** if used in the third trimester. (See Helpful Hints below.)

Helpful Hints and Reminders: Each pregnancy risk category (**A**, **B**, **C**, **D**, or **X**) is explained on the last page of this section.

1. Ibuprofen is a member of the non-steroidal, anti-inflammatory family of drugs, or NSAIDs. Members of this family of drugs should not be used during the third trimester of pregnancy (last 12 weeks) unless specifically prescribed by a clinician. See the Appendix for "Non-Steroidal, Anti-Inflammatory Drugs (NSAIDs) in Pregnancy," which describes the serious problems these drugs may cause for unborn babies when taken in the third trimester of pregnancy.

2. Women attempting to conceive should not use any NSAID, including Ibuprofen, because of the findings in animals that these drugs may block implantation of the early embryo in the wall of the uterus, in effect preventing pregnancy.

Remember: All pregnancies have a background risk of 3% or more for a serious birth defect, even when mom doesn't take a drug of any kind. If you are pregnant or planning a pregnancy, always let your healthcare provider know before taking any drug, prescription or non-prescription, or herbal remedy.

Advil® Multi-Symptom Cold Caplets

Active Ingredient:	Pregnancy Risk Category:
Chlorpheniramine maleate	B
Pseudoephedrine Hcl	C

(continued)

Ibuprofen	Ibuprofen has two pregnancy risk categories: **B** when used in the first or second trimesters of pregnancy; **D** if used in the third trimester. (See Helpful Hints below.)

Helpful Hints and Reminders: Each pregnancy risk category (**A**, **B**, **C**, **D**, or **X**) is explained on the last page of this section.

1. Ibuprofen is a member of the non-steroidal, anti-inflammatory family of drugs, or NSAIDs. Members of this family of drugs should not be used during the third trimester of pregnancy (last 12 weeks) unless specifically prescribed by a clinician. See the Appendix for "Non-Steroidal, Anti-Inflammatory Drugs (NSAIDs) in Pregnancy," which describes the serious problems these drugs may cause for unborn babies when taken in the third trimester of pregnancy.

2. Women attempting to conceive should not use any NSAID, including Ibuprofen, because of the findings in animals that these drugs may block implantation of the early embryo in the wall of the uterus, in effect preventing pregnancy.

Remember: All pregnancies have a background risk of 3% or more for a serious birth defect, even when mom doesn't take a drug of any kind. If you are pregnant or planning a pregnancy, always let your healthcare provider know before taking any drug, prescription or non-prescription, or herbal remedy.

Afrin® 12 Hour Spray, Sinus

Active Ingredient:	Pregnancy Risk Category:
Oxymetazoline hydrochloride	C

Helpful Hints and Reminders: Each pregnancy risk category (**A**, **B**, **C**, **D**, or **X**) is explained on the last page of this section.

Remember: All pregnancies have a background risk of 3% or more for a serious birth defect, even when mom doesn't take a drug of any kind. If you are pregnant or planning a pregnancy, always let your healthcare

provider know before taking any drug, prescription or non-prescription, or herbal remedy.

Afrin® All Night No Drip, Nasal Spray

Active Ingredient:	Pregnancy Risk Category:
Oxymetazoline hydrochloride	C

Helpful Hints and Reminders: Each pregnancy risk category (**A**, **B**, **C**, **D**, or **X**) is explained on the last page of this section.

Remember: All pregnancies have a background risk of 3% or more for a serious birth defect, even when mom doesn't take a drug of any kind. If you are pregnant or planning a pregnancy, always let your healthcare provider know before taking any drug, prescription or non-prescription, or herbal remedy.

Afrin® No Drip 12 Hour Pump Mist, Extra Moisturizing

Active Ingredient:	Pregnancy Risk Category:
Oxymetazoline hydrochloride	C

Helpful Hints and Reminders: Each pregnancy risk category (**A**, **B**, **C**, **D**, or **X**) is explained on the last page of this section.

Remember: All pregnancies have a background risk of 3% or more for a serious birth defect, even when mom doesn't take a drug of any kind. If you are pregnant or planning a pregnancy, always let your healthcare provider know before taking any drug, prescription or non-prescription, or herbal remedy.

Afrin® No Drip 12 Hour Pump Mist, Severe Congestion

Active Ingredient:	Pregnancy Risk Category:
Oxymetazoline hydrochloride	C

Helpful Hints and Reminders: Each pregnancy risk category (**A**, **B**, **C**, **D**, or **X**) is explained on the last page of this section.

Remember: All pregnancies have a background risk of 3% or more for a serious birth defect, even when mom doesn't take a drug of any kind. If you are pregnant or planning a pregnancy, always let your healthcare provider know before taking any drug, prescription or non-prescription, or herbal remedy.

Afrin® No Drip Original 12 Hour Pump Mist

Active Ingredient:	Pregnancy Risk Category:
Oxymetazoline hydrochloride	C

Helpful Hints and Reminders: Each pregnancy risk category (**A**, **B**, **C**, **D**, or **X**) is explained on the last page of this section.

Remember: All pregnancies have a background risk of 3% or more for a serious birth defect, even when mom doesn't take a drug of any kind. If you are pregnant or planning a pregnancy, always let your healthcare provider know before taking any drug, prescription or non-prescription, or herbal remedy.

Alka-Seltzer Plus® Cherry Burst Cold Formula

Active Ingredient:	Pregnancy Risk Category:
Chlorpheniramine maleate	B
Phenylephrine bitartrate	C
Aspirin	Aspirin has two pregnancy risk categories: **C** when used in the first or second trimesters of pregnancy; **D** if used in the third trimester. (See Helpful Hints below.)

Helpful Hints and Reminders: Each pregnancy risk category (**A**, **B**, **C**, **D**, or **X**) is explained on the last page of this section.

1. Aspirin is a member of the non-steroidal, anti-inflammatory family of drugs, or NSAIDs. Members of this family of drugs should not be used during the third trimester of pregnancy (last 12 weeks) unless specifically prescribed by a clinician. See the Appendix for "Non-Steroidal, Anti-Inflammatory Drugs (NSAIDs) in Pregnancy,"

which describes the serious problems these drugs may cause for unborn babies when taken in the third trimester of pregnancy.

2. Women attempting to conceive should not use any NSAID, including aspirin, because of the findings in animals that these drugs may block implantation of the early embryo in the wall of the uterus, in effect preventing pregnancy.

Remember: All pregnancies have a background risk of 3% or more for a serious birth defect, even when mom doesn't take a drug of any kind. If you are pregnant or planning a pregnancy, always let your healthcare provider know before taking any drug, prescription or non-prescription, or herbal remedy.

Alka-Seltzer Plus® Cold & Cough Formula Liquid Gels

Active Ingredient:	Pregnancy Risk Category:
Acetaminophen	B
Chlorpheniramine maleate	B
Dextromethorphan Hbr	C
Phenylephrine Hcl	C

Helpful Hints and Reminders: Each pregnancy risk category (**A**, **B**, **C**, **D**, or **X**) is explained on the last page of this section.

Remember: All pregnancies have a background risk of 3% or more for a serious birth defect, even when mom doesn't take a drug of any kind. If you are pregnant or planning a pregnancy, always let your healthcare provider know before taking any drug, prescription or non-prescription, or herbal remedy.

Alka-Seltzer Plus® Cold & Cough Formula Tablets

Active Ingredient:	Pregnancy Risk Category:
Chlorpheniramine maleate	B
Dextromethorphan Hbr	C

(continued)

Phenylephrine bitartrate	C
Aspirin	Aspirin has two pregnancy risk categories: **C** when used in the first or second trimesters of pregnancy; **D** if used in the third trimester. (See Helpful Hints below.)

Helpful Hints and Reminders: Each pregnancy risk category (**A**, **B**, **C**, **D**, or **X**) is explained on the last page of this section.

1. Aspirin is a member of the non-steroidal, anti-inflammatory family of drugs, or NSAIDs. Members of this family of drugs should not be used during the third trimester of pregnancy (last 12 weeks) unless specifically prescribed by a clinician. See the Appendix for "Non-Steroidal, Anti-Inflammatory Drugs (NSAIDs) in Pregnancy," which describes the serious problems these drugs may cause for unborn babies when taken in the third trimester of pregnancy.

2. Women attempting to conceive should not use any NSAID, including aspirin, because of the findings in animals that these drugs may block implantation of the early embryo in the wall of the uterus, in effect preventing pregnancy.

Remember: All pregnancies have a background risk of 3% or more for a serious birth defect, even when mom doesn't take a drug of any kind. If you are pregnant or planning a pregnancy, always let your healthcare provider know before taking any drug, prescription or non-prescription, or herbal remedy.

Alka-Seltzer Plus® Day & Night Cold Formula Liquid Gels

Active Ingredient:	Pregnancy Risk Category:
Day Cold:	
Acetaminophen	B
Dextromethorphan Hbr	C

(continued)

Alka-Seltzer Plus® Day & Night Cold Formula Tablets

Phenylephrine Hcl	C
Night Cold:	
Acetaminophen	B
Dextromethorphan Hbr	C
Doxylamine succinate	A
Phenylephrine Hcl	C

Helpful Hints and Reminders: Each pregnancy risk category (**A**, **B**, **C**, **D**, or **X**) is explained on the last page of this section.

Remember: All pregnancies have a background risk of 3% or more for a serious birth defect, even when mom doesn't take a drug of any kind. If you are pregnant or planning a pregnancy, always let your healthcare provider know before taking any drug, prescription or non-prescription, or herbal remedy.

· ·

Alka-Seltzer Plus® Day & Night Cold Formula Tablets

Active Ingredient:	Pregnancy Risk Category:
Day Cold:	
Dextromethorphan Hbr	C
Phenylephrine bitartrate	C
Aspirin	Aspirin has two pregnancy risk categories: **B** when used in the first or second trimesters of pregnancy; **D** if used in the third trimester. (See Helpful Hints on the next page.)
Night Cold:	
Dextromethorphan Hbr	C
Doxylamine succinate	A
Phenylephrine bitartrate	C

(*continued*)

| Aspirin | Aspirin has two pregnancy risk categories: **B** when used in the first or second trimesters of pregnancy; **D** if used in the third trimester. (See Helpful Hints below.) |

Helpful Hints and Reminders: Each pregnancy risk category (**A**, **B**, **C**, **D**, or **X**) is explained on the last page of this section.

1. Aspirin is a member of the non-steroidal, anti-inflammatory family of drugs, or NSAIDs. Members of this family of drugs should not be used during the third trimester of pregnancy (last 12 weeks) unless specifically prescribed by a clinician. See the Appendix for "Non-Steroidal, Anti-Inflammatory Drugs (NSAIDs) in Pregnancy," which describes the serious problems these drugs may cause for unborn babies when taken in the third trimester of pregnancy.

2. Women attempting to conceive should not use any NSAID, including aspirin, because of the findings in animals that these drugs may block implantation of the early embryo in the wall of the uterus, in effect preventing pregnancy.

Remember: All pregnancies have a background risk of 3% or more for a serious birth defect, even when mom doesn't take a drug of any kind. If you are pregnant or planning a pregnancy, always let your healthcare provider know before taking any drug, prescription or non-prescription, or herbal remedy.

Alka-Seltzer Plus® Day Non-Drowsy Cold Formula

Active Ingredient:	Pregnancy Risk Category:
Acetaminophen	B
Dextromethorphan Hbr	C
Phenylephrine Hcl	C

Helpful Hints and Reminders: Each pregnancy risk category (**A**, **B**, **C**, **D**, or **X**) is explained on the last page of this section.

Remember: All pregnancies have a background risk of 3% or more for a serious birth defect, even when mom doesn't take a drug of any kind. If you are pregnant or planning a pregnancy, always let your healthcare provider know before taking any drug, prescription or non-prescription, or herbal remedy.

Alka-Seltzer Plus® Fast Crystal Packs

Active Ingredient:	Pregnancy Risk Category:
Acetaminophen	B
Chlorpheniramine maleate	B
Phenylephrine	C

Helpful Hints and Reminders: Each pregnancy risk category (**A**, **B**, **C**, **D**, or **X**) is explained on the last page of this section.

Remember: All pregnancies have a background risk of 3% or more for a serious birth defect, even when mom doesn't take a drug of any kind. If you are pregnant or planning a pregnancy, always let your healthcare provider know before taking any drug, prescription or non-prescription, or herbal remedy.

Alka-Seltzer Plus® Flu Formula

Active Ingredient:	Pregnancy Risk Category:
Chlorpheniramine maleate	B
Dextromethorphan Hbr	C
Aspirin	Aspirin has two pregnancy risk categories: **C** when used in the first or second trimesters of pregnancy; **D** if used in the third trimester. (See Helpful Hints below.)

Helpful Hints and Reminders: Each pregnancy risk category (**A**, **B**, **C**, **D**, or **X**) is explained on the last page of this section.

1. Aspirin is a member of the non-steroidal, anti-inflammatory family of drugs, or NSAIDs. Members of this family of drugs should not be used during the third trimester of pregnancy (last 12 weeks)

unless specifically prescribed by a clinician. See the Appendix for "Non-Steroidal, Anti-Inflammatory Drugs (NSAIDs) in Pregnancy," which describes the serious problems these drugs may cause for unborn babies when taken in the third trimester of pregnancy.

2. Women attempting to conceive should not use any NSAID, including aspirin, because of the findings in animals that these drugs may block implantation of the early embryo in the wall of the uterus, in effect preventing pregnancy.

Remember: All pregnancies have a background risk of 3% or more for a serious birth defect, even when mom doesn't take a drug of any kind. If you are pregnant or planning a pregnancy, always let your healthcare provider know before taking any drug, prescription or non-prescription, or herbal remedy.

Alka-Seltzer Plus® Mucus & Congestion Liquid Gels

Active Ingredient:	Pregnancy Risk Category:
Dextromethorphan Hbr	C
Guaifenesin	C

Helpful Hints and Reminders: Each pregnancy risk category (**A**, **B**, **C**, **D**, or **X**) is explained on the last page of this section.

Remember: All pregnancies have a background risk of 3% or more for a serious birth defect, even when mom doesn't take a drug of any kind. If you are pregnant or planning a pregnancy, always let your healthcare provider know before taking any drug, prescription or non-prescription, or herbal remedy.

Alka-Seltzer Plus® Night Cold Formula

Active Ingredient:	Pregnancy Risk Category:
Doxylamine succinate	A
Dextromethorphan Hbr	C
Phenylephrine bitartrate	C

(continued)

| Aspirin | Aspirin has two pregnancy risk categories: **C** when used in the first or second trimesters of pregnancy; **D** if used in the third trimester. (See Helpful Hints below.) |

Helpful Hints and Reminders: Each pregnancy risk category (**A**, **B**, **C**, **D**, or **X**) is explained on the last page of this section.

1. Aspirin is a member of the non-steroidal, anti-inflammatory family of drugs, or NSAIDs. Members of this family of drugs should not be used during the third trimester of pregnancy (last 12 weeks) unless specifically prescribed by a clinician. See the Appendix for "Non-Steroidal, Anti-Inflammatory Drugs (NSAIDs) in Pregnancy," which describes the serious problems these drugs may cause for unborn babies when taken in the third trimester of pregnancy.

2. Women attempting to conceive should not use any NSAID, including aspirin, because of the findings in animals that these drugs may block implantation of the early embryo in the wall of the uterus, in effect preventing pregnancy.

Remember: All pregnancies have a background risk of 3% or more for a serious birth defect, even when mom doesn't take a drug of any kind. If you are pregnant or planning a pregnancy, always let your healthcare provider know before taking any drug, prescription or non-prescription, or herbal remedy.

Alka-Seltzer Plus® Night Cold Formula Liquid Gels

Active Ingredient:	Pregnancy Risk Category:
Acetaminophen	B
Doxylamine succinate	A
Dextromethorphan Hbr	C
Phenylephrine Hcl	C

Helpful Hints and Reminders: Each pregnancy risk category (**A**, **B**, **C**, **D**, or **X**) is explained on the last page of this section.

Remember: All pregnancies have a background risk of 3% or more for a serious birth defect, even when mom doesn't take a drug of any kind. If you are pregnant or planning a pregnancy, always let your healthcare provider know before taking any drug, prescription or non-prescription, or herbal remedy.

Alka-Seltzer Plus® Orange Zest Cold Formula

Active Ingredient:	Pregnancy Risk Category:
Chlorpheniramine maleate	B
Phenylephrine bitartrate	C
Aspirin	Aspirin has two pregnancy risk categories: **C** when used in the first or second trimesters of pregnancy; **D** if used in the third trimester. (See Helpful Hints below.)

Helpful Hints and Reminders: Each pregnancy risk category (**A**, **B**, **C**, **D**, or **X**) is explained on the last page of this section.

1. Aspirin is a member of the non-steroidal, anti-inflammatory family of drugs, or NSAIDs. Members of this family of drugs should not be used during the third trimester of pregnancy (last 12 weeks) unless specifically prescribed by a clinician. See the Appendix for "Non-Steroidal, Anti-Inflammatory Drugs (NSAIDs) in Pregnancy," which describes the serious problems these drugs may cause for unborn babies when taken in the third trimester of pregnancy.

2. Women attempting to conceive should not use any NSAID, including aspirin, because of the findings in animals that these drugs may block implantation of the early embryo in the wall of the uterus, in effect preventing pregnancy.

Remember: All pregnancies have a background risk of 3% or more for a serious birth defect, even when mom doesn't take a drug of any kind.

Alka-Seltzer Plus® Sparkling Original Cold Formula   **53**

If you are pregnant or planning a pregnancy, always let your healthcare provider know before taking any drug, prescription or non-prescription, or herbal remedy.

Alka-Seltzer Plus® Sparkling Original Cold Formula

Active Ingredient:	Pregnancy Risk Category:
Chlorpheniramine maleate	**B**
Phenylephrine bitartrate	**C**
Aspirin	Aspirin has two pregnancy risk categories: **C** when used in the first or second trimesters of pregnancy; **D** if used in the third trimester. (See Helpful Hints below.)

Helpful Hints and Reminders: Each pregnancy risk category (**A**, **B**, **C**, **D**, or **X**) is explained on the last page of this section.

1. Aspirin is a member of the non-steroidal, anti-inflammatory family of drugs, or NSAIDs. Members of this family of drugs should not be used during the third trimester of pregnancy (last 12 weeks) unless specifically prescribed by a clinician. See the Appendix for "Non-Steroidal, Anti-Inflammatory Drugs (NSAIDs) in Pregnancy," which describes the serious problems these drugs may cause for unborn babies when taken in the third trimester of pregnancy.

2. Women attempting to conceive should not use any NSAID, including aspirin, because of the findings in animals that these drugs may block implantation of the early embryo in the wall of the uterus, in effect preventing pregnancy.

Remember: All pregnancies have a background risk of 3% or more for a serious birth defect, even when mom doesn't take a drug of any kind. If you are pregnant or planning a pregnancy, always let your healthcare provider know before taking any drug, prescription or non-prescription, or herbal remedy.

Benylin® All-in-One® Cold and Flu Caplets

Active Ingredient:	Pregnancy Risk Category:
Dextromethorphan Hbr	C
Pseudoephedrine Hcl	C
Guaifenesin	C
Acetaminophen	B

Helpful Hints and Reminders: Each pregnancy risk category (**A**, **B**, **C**, **D**, or **X**) is explained on the last page of this section.

Remember: All pregnancies have a background risk of 3% or more for a serious birth defect, even when mom doesn't take a drug of any kind. If you are pregnant or planning a pregnancy, always let your healthcare provider know before taking any drug, prescription or non-prescription, or herbal remedy.

Benylin® All-in-One® Cold and Flu Night Caplets

Active Ingredient:	Pregnancy Risk Category:
Acetaminophen	B
Phenylephrine Hcl	C
Diphenhydramine Hcl	B

Helpful Hints and Reminders: Each pregnancy risk category (**A**, **B**, **C**, **D**, or **X**) is explained on the last page of this section.

Remember: All pregnancies have a background risk of 3% or more for a serious birth defect, even when mom doesn't take a drug of any kind. If you are pregnant or planning a pregnancy, always let your healthcare provider know before taking any drug, prescription or non-prescription, or herbal remedy.

Benylin® All-in-One® Cold and Flu Syrup

Active Ingredient:	Pregnancy Risk Category:
Dextromethorphan Hbr	C
Pseudoephedrine Hcl	C
Guaifenesin	C
Acetaminophen	B

Helpful Hints and Reminders: Each pregnancy risk category (**A**, **B**, **C**, **D**, or **X**) is explained on the last page of this section.

Remember: All pregnancies have a background risk of 3% or more for a serious birth defect, even when mom doesn't take a drug of any kind. If you are pregnant or planning a pregnancy, always let your healthcare provider know before taking any drug, prescription or non-prescription, or herbal remedy.

Benylin® All-in-One® Extra Strength Cold & Flu Nighttime Syrup

Active Ingredient:	Pregnancy Risk Category:
Chlorpheniramine maleate	B
Dextromethorphan Hbr	C
Pseudoephedrine Hcl	C
Guaifenesin	C
Acetaminophen	B

Helpful Hints and Reminders: Each pregnancy risk category (**A**, **B**, **C**, **D**, or **X**) is explained on the last page of this section.

Remember: All pregnancies have a background risk of 3% or more for a serious birth defect, even when mom doesn't take a drug of any kind. If you are pregnant or planning a pregnancy, always let your healthcare provider know before taking any drug, prescription or non-prescription, or herbal remedy.

Benylin® Cold & Flu with Codeine

Active Ingredient:	Pregnancy Risk Category:
Pseudoephedrine Hcl	C
Guaifenesin	C
Codeine phosphate	C, but risk factor **D** if used for prolonged periods in pregnancy or in high doses near term. (See Helpful Hints below.)

Helpful Hints and Reminders: Each pregnancy risk category (**A**, **B**, **C**, **D**, or **X**) is explained on the last page of this section.

1. Excessive fetal exposure to codeine, especially near term, may cause respiratory depression in newborns at delivery.

Remember: All pregnancies have a background risk of 3% or more for a serious birth defect, even when mom doesn't take a drug of any kind. If you are pregnant or planning a pregnancy, always let your healthcare provider know before taking any drug, prescription or non-prescription, or herbal remedy.

Benylin® Cold & Sinus Day/Night Caplets

Active Ingredient:	Pregnancy Risk Category:
Phenylephrine Hcl	C
Acetaminophen	B

Helpful Hints and Reminders: Each pregnancy risk category (**A**, **B**, **C**, **D**, or **X**) is explained on the last page of this section.

Remember: All pregnancies have a background risk of 3% or more for a serious birth defect, even when mom doesn't take a drug of any kind. If you are pregnant or planning a pregnancy, always let your healthcare provider know before taking any drug, prescription or non-prescription, or herbal remedy.

Benylin® Cold & Sinus Plus Caplets

Active Ingredient:	Pregnancy Risk Category:
Phenylephrine Hcl	C
Acetaminophen	B
Chlorpheniramine maleate	B

Helpful Hints and Reminders: Each pregnancy risk category (**A**, **B**, **C**, **D**, or **X**) is explained on the last page of this section.

Remember: All pregnancies have a background risk of 3% or more for a serious birth defect, even when mom doesn't take a drug of any kind. If you are pregnant or planning a pregnancy, always let your healthcare provider know before taking any drug, prescription or non-prescription, or herbal remedy.

Benylin® DM® Tickly Throat & Cough

Active Ingredient:	Pregnancy Risk Category:
Dextromethorphan Hbr	C

Helpful Hints and Reminders: Each pregnancy risk category (**A**, **B**, **C**, **D**, or **X**) is explained on the last page of this section.

Remember: All pregnancies have a background risk of 3% or more for a serious birth defect, even when mom doesn't take a drug of any kind. If you are pregnant or planning a pregnancy, always let your healthcare provider know before taking any drug, prescription or non-prescription, or herbal remedy.

Benylin® DM-D-E® Cough & Chest Congestion with Warming Sensation

Active Ingredient:	Pregnancy Risk Category:
Dextromethorphan Hbr	C
Pseudoephedrine Hcl	C
Guaifenesin	C

Helpful Hints and Reminders: Each pregnancy risk category (**A**, **B**, **C**, **D**, or **X**) is explained on the last page of this section.

Remember: All pregnancies have a background risk of 3% or more for a serious birth defect, even when mom doesn't take a drug of any kind. If you are pregnant or planning a pregnancy, always let your healthcare provider know before taking any drug, prescription or non-prescription, or herbal remedy.

Benylin® DM-D-E® Extra Strength Chest Cough and Cold

Active Ingredient:	Pregnancy Risk Category:
Dextromethorphan Hbr	C
Pseudoephedrine Hcl	C
Guaifenesin	C
Menthol	**Risk is undetermined**, but thought to be small, according to the Illinois Teratogen Information Service (ITIS).

Helpful Hints and Reminders: Each pregnancy risk category (**A**, **B**, **C**, **D**, or **X**) is explained on the last page of this section.

Remember: All pregnancies have a background risk of 3% or more for a serious birth defect, even when mom doesn't take a drug of any kind. If you are pregnant or planning a pregnancy, always let your healthcare provider know before taking any drug, prescription or non-prescription, or herbal remedy.

Benylin® DM-D-E-A® Cough & Cold with Warming Sensation

Active Ingredient:	Pregnancy Risk Category:
Dextromethorphan Hbr	C
Pseudoephedrine Hcl	C
Acetaminophen	B

Helpful Hints and Reminders: Each pregnancy risk category (**A**, **B**, **C**, **D**, or **X**) is explained on the last page of this section.

Remember: All pregnancies have a background risk of 3% or more for a serious birth defect, even when mom doesn't take a drug of any kind. If you are pregnant or planning a pregnancy, always let your healthcare provider know before taking any drug, prescription or non-prescription, or herbal remedy.

Benylin® DM-E® Extra Strength Chest Cough & Cold

Active Ingredient:	Pregnancy Risk Category:
Dextromethorphan Hbr	C
Guaifenesin	C
Menthol	**Risk is undetermined**, but thought to be small, according to the Illinois Teratogen Information Service (ITIS).

Helpful Hints and Reminders: Each pregnancy risk category (**A**, **B**, **C**, **D**, or **X**) is explained on the last page of this section.

Remember: All pregnancies have a background risk of 3% or more for a serious birth defect, even when mom doesn't take a drug of any kind. If you are pregnant or planning a pregnancy, always let your healthcare provider know before taking any drug, prescription or non-prescription, or herbal remedy.

Benylin® E® Extra Strength Chest Congestion

Active Ingredient:	Pregnancy Risk Category:
Guaifenesin	C
Menthol	**Risk is undetermined**, but thought to be small, according to the Illinois Teratogen Information Service (ITIS).

Helpful Hints and Reminders: Each pregnancy risk category (**A**, **B**, **C**, **D**, or **X**) is explained on the last page of this section.

Remember: All pregnancies have a background risk of 3% or more for a serious birth defect, even when mom doesn't take a drug of any kind. If you are pregnant or planning a pregnancy, always let your healthcare provider know before taking any drug, prescription or non-prescription, or herbal remedy.

Benylin® E® Menthol Mucous & Phlegm Relief

Active Ingredient:	Pregnancy Risk Category:
Guaifenesin	C
Menthol	**Risk is undetermined**, but thought to be small, according to the Illinois Teratogen Information Service (ITIS).

Helpful Hints and Reminders: Each pregnancy risk category (**A**, **B**, **C**, **D**, or **X**) is explained on the last page of this section.

Remember: All pregnancies have a background risk of 3% or more for a serious birth defect, even when mom doesn't take a drug of any kind. If you are pregnant or planning a pregnancy, always let your healthcare provider know before taking any drug, prescription or non-prescription, or herbal remedy.

Benylin® Extra Strength Mucous & Phlegm Relief Plus Cough Control

Active Ingredient:	Pregnancy Risk Category:
Dextromethorphan Hbr	C
Guaifenesin	C
Menthol	**Risk is undetermined**, but thought to be small, according to the Illinois Teratogen Information Service (ITIS).

Buckley's® Cough Mixture

Helpful Hints and Reminders: Each pregnancy risk category (**A**, **B**, **C**, **D**, or **X**) is explained on the last page of this section.

Remember: All pregnancies have a background risk of 3% or more for a serious birth defect, even when mom doesn't take a drug of any kind. If you are pregnant or planning a pregnancy, always let your healthcare provider know before taking any drug, prescription or non-prescription, or herbal remedy.

Buckley's® Chest Congestion Mixture

Active Ingredient:	Pregnancy Risk Category:
Guaifenesin	C

Helpful Hints and Reminders: Each pregnancy risk category (**A**, **B**, **C**, **D**, or **X**) is explained on the last page of this section.

Remember: All pregnancies have a background risk of 3% or more for a serious birth defect, even when mom doesn't take a drug of any kind. If you are pregnant or planning a pregnancy, always let your healthcare provider know before taking any drug, prescription or non-prescription, or herbal remedy.

Buckley's® Cough Mixture

Active Ingredient:	Pregnancy Risk Category:
Dextromethorphan	C

Helpful Hints and Reminders: Each pregnancy risk category (**A**, **B**, **C**, **D**, or **X**) is explained on the last page of this section.

Remember: All pregnancies have a background risk of 3% or more for a serious birth defect, even when mom doesn't take a drug of any kind. If you are pregnant or planning a pregnancy, always let your healthcare provider know before taking any drug, prescription or non-prescription, or herbal remedy.

Comtrex® Maximum Strength Day/Night Cold & Cough Caplets

Active Ingredient:	Pregnancy Risk Category:
Acetaminophen	B
Chlorpheniramine maleate	B
Dextromethorphan	C
Phenylephrine	C

Helpful Hints and Reminders: Each pregnancy risk category (**A**, **B**, **C**, **D**, or **X**) is explained on the last page of this section.

Remember: All pregnancies have a background risk of 3% or more for a serious birth defect, even when mom doesn't take a drug of any kind. If you are pregnant or planning a pregnancy, always let your healthcare provider know before taking any drug, prescription or non-prescription, or herbal remedy.

Comtrex® Maximum Strength Non-Drowsy Cold & Cough

Active Ingredient:	Pregnancy Risk Category:
Acetaminophen	B
Dextromethorphan	C
Phenylephrine	C

Helpful Hints and Reminders: Each pregnancy risk category (**A**, **B**, **C**, **D**, or **X**) is explained on the last page of this section.

Remember: All pregnancies have a background risk of 3% or more for a serious birth defect, even when mom doesn't take a drug of any kind. If you are pregnant or planning a pregnancy, always let your healthcare provider know before taking any drug, prescription or non-prescription, or herbal remedy.

Contac® Cold + Flu Day & Night Dual Formula Pack Caplets

Active Ingredient:	Pregnancy Risk Category:
Day Caplet:	
Acetaminophen	B
Phenylephrine Hcl	C
Night Caplet:	
Acetaminophen	B
Phenylephrine Hcl	C
Chlorpheniramine maleate	B

Helpful Hints and Reminders: Each pregnancy risk category (**A**, **B**, **C**, **D**, or **X**) is explained on the last page of this section.

Remember: All pregnancies have a background risk of 3% or more for a serious birth defect, even when mom doesn't take a drug of any kind. If you are pregnant or planning a pregnancy, always let your healthcare provider know before taking any drug, prescription or non-prescription, or herbal remedy.

Contac® Cold + Flu Maximum Strength Caplets

Active Ingredient:	Pregnancy Risk Category:
Acetaminophen	B
Chlorpheniramine maleate	B
Phenylephrine Hcl	C

Helpful Hints and Reminders: Each pregnancy risk category (**A**, **B**, **C**, **D**, or **X**) is explained on the last page of this section.

Remember: All pregnancies have a background risk of 3% or more for a serious birth defect, even when mom doesn't take a drug of any kind. If you are pregnant or planning a pregnancy, always let your healthcare provider know before taking any drug, prescription or non-prescription, or herbal remedy.

Contac® Cold + Flu Non-Drowsy Maximum Strength Caplets

Active Ingredient:	Pregnancy Risk Category:
Acetaminophen	B
Phenylephrine Hcl	C

Helpful Hints and Reminders: Each pregnancy risk category (**A**, **B**, **C**, **D**, or **X**) is explained on the last page of this section.

Remember: All pregnancies have a background risk of 3% or more for a serious birth defect, even when mom doesn't take a drug of any kind. If you are pregnant or planning a pregnancy, always let your healthcare provider know before taking any drug, prescription or non-prescription, or herbal remedy.

Coricidin® HBP Chest Congestion & Cough

Active Ingredient:	Pregnancy Risk Category:
Dextromethorphan Hbr	C
Guaifenesin	C

Helpful Hints and Reminders: Each pregnancy risk category (**A**, **B**, **C**, **D**, or **X**) is explained on the last page of this section.

Remember: All pregnancies have a background risk of 3% or more for a serious birth defect, even when mom doesn't take a drug of any kind. If you are pregnant or planning a pregnancy, always let your healthcare provider know before taking any drug, prescription or non-prescription, or herbal remedy.

Coricidin® HBP Cold & Flu

Active Ingredient:	Pregnancy Risk Category:
Acetaminophen	B
Chlorpheniramine maleate	B

Helpful Hints and Reminders: Each pregnancy risk category (**A**, **B**, **C**, **D**, or **X**) is explained on the last page of this section.

Remember: All pregnancies have a background risk of 3% or more for a serious birth defect, even when mom doesn't take a drug of any kind. If you are pregnant or planning a pregnancy, always let your healthcare provider know before taking any drug, prescription or non-prescription, or herbal remedy.

Coricidin® HBP Cough & Cold

Active Ingredient:	Pregnancy Risk Category:
Chlorpheniramine maleate	B
Dextromethorphan Hbr	C

Helpful Hints and Reminders: Each pregnancy risk category (**A**, **B**, **C**, **D**, or **X**) is explained on the last page of this section.

Remember: All pregnancies have a background risk of 3% or more for a serious birth defect, even when mom doesn't take a drug of any kind. If you are pregnant or planning a pregnancy, always let your healthcare provider know before taking any drug, prescription or non-prescription, or herbal remedy.

Coricidin® HBP Day & Night Multi-Symptom Cold

Active Ingredient:	Pregnancy Risk Category:
Daytime Softgel:	
Dextromethorphan Hbr	C
Guaifenesin	C
Nighttime Softgel:	
Acetaminophen	B
Chlorpheniramine maleate	B
Dextromethorphan Hbr	C

Helpful Hints and Reminders: Each pregnancy risk category (**A**, **B**, **C**, **D**, or **X**) is explained on the last page of this section.

Remember: All pregnancies have a background risk of 3% or more for a serious birth defect, even when mom doesn't take a drug of any kind. If you are pregnant or planning a pregnancy, always let your healthcare provider know before taking any drug, prescription or non-prescription, or herbal remedy.

Coricidin® HBP Maximum Strength Flu

Active Ingredient:	Pregnancy Risk Category:
Acetaminophen	B
Chlorpheniramine maleate	B
Dextromethorphan Hbr	C

Helpful Hints and Reminders: Each pregnancy risk category (**A**, **B**, **C**, **D**, or **X**) is explained on the last page of this section.

Remember: All pregnancies have a background risk of 3% or more for a serious birth defect, even when mom doesn't take a drug of any kind. If you are pregnant or planning a pregnancy, always let your healthcare provider know before taking any drug, prescription or non-prescription, or herbal remedy.

Coricidin® HPB Nighttime Multi-Symptom Cold

Active Ingredient:	Pregnancy Risk Category:
Acetaminophen	B
Doxylamine succinate	A
Dextromethorphan Hbr	C

Helpful Hints and Reminders: Each pregnancy risk category (**A**, **B**, **C**, **D**, or **X**) is explained on the last page of this section.

Remember: All pregnancies have a background risk of 3% or more for a serious birth defect, even when mom doesn't take a drug of any kind.

If you are pregnant or planning a pregnancy, always let your healthcare provider know before taking any drug, prescription or non-prescription, or herbal remedy.

CVS® Chest Congestion Relief PE Tablets

Active Ingredient:	Pregnancy Risk Category:
Guaifenesin	C
Phenylephrine Hcl	C

Helpful Hints and Reminders: Each pregnancy risk category (**A**, **B**, **C**, **D**, or **X**) is explained on the last page of this section.

Remember: All pregnancies have a background risk of 3% or more for a serious birth defect, even when mom doesn't take a drug of any kind. If you are pregnant or planning a pregnancy, always let your healthcare provider know before taking any drug, prescription or non-prescription, or herbal remedy.

CVS® Cold & Flu BP Tablets

Active Ingredient:	Pregnancy Risk Category:
Acetaminophen	B
Chlorpheniramine maleate	B

Helpful Hints and Reminders: Each pregnancy risk category (**A**, **B**, **C**, **D**, or **X**) is explained on the last page of this section.

Remember: All pregnancies have a background risk of 3% or more for a serious birth defect, even when mom doesn't take a drug of any kind. If you are pregnant or planning a pregnancy, always let your healthcare provider know before taking any drug, prescription or non-prescription, or herbal remedy.

CVS® Flu & Severe Cold Nighttime Cherry Flavor

Active Ingredient:	Pregnancy Risk Category:
Acetaminophen	B
Diphenhydramine Hcl	B
Phenylephrine	C

Helpful Hints and Reminders: Each pregnancy risk category (**A**, **B**, **C**, **D**, or **X**) is explained on the last page of this section.

Remember: All pregnancies have a background risk of 3% or more for a serious birth defect, even when mom doesn't take a drug of any kind. If you are pregnant or planning a pregnancy, always let your healthcare provider know before taking any drug, prescription or non-prescription, or herbal remedy.

CVS® Nighttime Cough & Severe Cold Packets Honey Lemon

Active Ingredient:	Pregnancy Risk Category:
Acetaminophen	B
Diphenhydramine Hcl	B
Phenylephrine Hcl	C

Helpful Hints and Reminders: Each pregnancy risk category (**A**, **B**, **C**, **D**, or **X**) is explained on the last page of this section.

Remember: All pregnancies have a background risk of 3% or more for a serious birth defect, even when mom doesn't take a drug of any kind. If you are pregnant or planning a pregnancy, always let your healthcare provider know before taking any drug, prescription or non-prescription, or herbal remedy.

CVS® Severe Cold Relief PE Multi-Symptom Caplets

Active Ingredient:	Pregnancy Risk Category:
Acetaminophen	B
Diphenhydramine Hcl	B
Phenylephrine Hcl	C

Helpful Hints and Reminders: Each pregnancy risk category (**A**, **B**, **C**, **D**, or **X**) is explained on the last page of this section.

Remember: All pregnancies have a background risk of 3% or more for a serious birth defect, even when mom doesn't take a drug of any kind. If you are pregnant or planning a pregnancy, always let your healthcare provider know before taking any drug, prescription or non-prescription, or herbal remedy.

CVS® Tussin Cough Formula Maximum Strength

Active Ingredient:	Pregnancy Risk Category:
Dextromethorphan Hbr	C

Helpful Hints and Reminders: Each pregnancy risk category (**A**, **B**, **C**, **D**, or **X**) is explained on the last page of this section.

Remember: All pregnancies have a background risk of 3% or more for a serious birth defect, even when mom doesn't take a drug of any kind. If you are pregnant or planning a pregnancy, always let your healthcare provider know before taking any drug, prescription or non-prescription, or herbal remedy.

CVS® Tussin DM Cough Suppressant

Active Ingredient:	Pregnancy Risk Category:
Dextromethorphan	C
Guaifenesin	C

Helpful Hints and Reminders: Each pregnancy risk category (**A**, **B**, **C**, **D**, or **X**) is explained on the last page of this section.

Remember: All pregnancies have a background risk of 3% or more for a serious birth defect, even when mom doesn't take a drug of any kind. If you are pregnant or planning a pregnancy, always let your healthcare provider know before taking any drug, prescription or non-prescription, or herbal remedy.

DayQuil® Cold & Flu Relief LiquiCaps

Active Ingredient:	Pregnancy Risk Category:
Acetaminophen	B
Phenylephrine Hcl	C
Dextromethorphan Hbr	C

Helpful Hints and Reminders: Each pregnancy risk category (**A**, **B**, **C**, **D**, or **X**) is explained on the last page of this section.

Remember: All pregnancies have a background risk of 3% or more for a serious birth defect, even when mom doesn't take a drug of any kind. If you are pregnant or planning a pregnancy, always let your healthcare provider know before taking any drug, prescription or non-prescription, or herbal remedy.

DayQuil® Cold & Flu Relief Liquid

Active Ingredient:	Pregnancy Risk Category:
Acetaminophen	B
Phenylephrine Hcl	C
Dextromethorphan Hbr	C

Helpful Hints and Reminders: Each pregnancy risk category (**A**, **B**, **C**, **D**, or **X**) is explained on the last page of this section.

Remember: All pregnancies have a background risk of 3% or more for a serious birth defect, even when mom doesn't take a drug of any kind.

DayQuil® Cough

If you are pregnant or planning a pregnancy, always let your healthcare provider know before taking any drug, prescription or non-prescription, or herbal remedy.

DayQuil® Cold & Flu Symptom Relief Plus Vitamin C

Active Ingredient:	Pregnancy Risk Category:
Acetaminophen	B
Phenylephrine Hcl	C
Dextromethorphan Hbr	C

Helpful Hints and Reminders: Each pregnancy risk category (**A**, **B**, **C**, **D**, or **X**) is explained on the last page of this section.

Remember: All pregnancies have a background risk of 3% or more for a serious birth defect, even when mom doesn't take a drug of any kind. If you are pregnant or planning a pregnancy, always let your healthcare provider know before taking any drug, prescription or non-prescription, or herbal remedy.

DayQuil® Cough

Active Ingredient:	Pregnancy Risk Category:
Dextromethorphan Hbr	C

Helpful Hints and Reminders: Each pregnancy risk category (**A**, **B**, **C**, **D**, or **X**) is explained on the last page of this section.

Remember: All pregnancies have a background risk of 3% or more for a serious birth defect, even when mom doesn't take a drug of any kind. If you are pregnant or planning a pregnancy, always let your healthcare provider know before taking any drug, prescription or non-prescription, or herbal remedy.

DayQuil® Mucus Control DM

Active Ingredient:	Pregnancy Risk Category:
Dextromethorphan	C
Guaifenesin	C

Helpful Hints and Reminders: Each pregnancy risk category (**A**, **B**, **C**, **D**, or **X**) is explained on the last page of this section.

Remember: All pregnancies have a background risk of 3% or more for a serious birth defect, even when mom doesn't take a drug of any kind. If you are pregnant or planning a pregnancy, always let your healthcare provider know before taking any drug, prescription or non-prescription, or herbal remedy.

DayQuil® Mucus Control Liquid

Active Ingredient:	Pregnancy Risk Category:
Guaifenesin	C

Helpful Hints and Reminders: Each pregnancy risk category (**A**, **B**, **C**, **D**, or **X**) is explained on the last page of this section.

Remember: All pregnancies have a background risk of 3% or more for a serious birth defect, even when mom doesn't take a drug of any kind. If you are pregnant or planning a pregnancy, always let your healthcare provider know before taking any drug, prescription or non-prescription, or herbal remedy.

Delsym® Liquid, Grape and Orange Flavors

Active Ingredient:	Pregnancy Risk Category:
Dextromethorphan Hbr	C

Helpful Hints and Reminders: Each pregnancy risk category (**A**, **B**, **C**, **D**, or **X**) is explained on the last page of this section.

Remember: All pregnancies have a background risk of 3% or more for a serious birth defect, even when mom doesn't take a drug of any kind.

If you are pregnant or planning a pregnancy, always let your healthcare provider know before taking any drug, prescription or non-prescription, or herbal remedy.

Diabetic Tussin® Cold & Flu Formula

Active Ingredient:	Pregnancy Risk Category:
Acetaminophen	B
Dextromethorphan Hbr	C
Diphenhydramine	B

Helpful Hints and Reminders: Each pregnancy risk category (**A**, **B**, **C**, **D**, or **X**) is explained on the last page of this section.

Remember: All pregnancies have a background risk of 3% or more for a serious birth defect, even when mom doesn't take a drug of any kind. If you are pregnant or planning a pregnancy, always let your healthcare provider know before taking any drug, prescription or non-prescription, or herbal remedy.

Diabetic Tussin® DM Cough Suppressant & Expectorant

Active Ingredient:	Pregnancy Risk Category:
Dextromethorphan Hbr	C
Guaifenesin	C

Helpful Hints and Reminders: Each pregnancy risk category (**A**, **B**, **C**, **D**, or **X**) is explained on the last page of this section.

Remember: All pregnancies have a background risk of 3% or more for a serious birth defect, even when mom doesn't take a drug of any kind. If you are pregnant or planning a pregnancy, always let your healthcare provider know before taking any drug, prescription or non-prescription, or herbal remedy.

Diabetic Tussin® DM Maximum Strength Cough Suppressant & Expectorant

Active Ingredient:	Pregnancy Risk Category:
Dextromethorphan Hbr	C
Guaifenesin	C

Helpful Hints and Reminders: Each pregnancy risk category (**A**, **B**, **C**, **D**, or **X**) is explained on the last page of this section.

Remember: All pregnancies have a background risk of 3% or more for a serious birth defect, even when mom doesn't take a drug of any kind. If you are pregnant or planning a pregnancy, always let your healthcare provider know before taking any drug, prescription or non-prescription, or herbal remedy.

Diabetic Tussin® EX 400 Expectorant Mucus Relief

Active Ingredient:	Pregnancy Risk Category:
Guaifenesin	C

Helpful Hints and Reminders: Each pregnancy risk category (**A**, **B**, **C**, **D**, or **X**) is explained on the last page of this section.

Remember: All pregnancies have a background risk of 3% or more for a serious birth defect, even when mom doesn't take a drug of any kind. If you are pregnant or planning a pregnancy, always let your healthcare provider know before taking any drug, prescription or non-prescription, or herbal remedy.

Diabetic Tussin® EX Expectorant

Active Ingredient:	Pregnancy Risk Category:
Guaifenesin	C

Helpful Hints and Reminders: Each pregnancy risk category (**A**, **B**, **C**, **D**, or **X**) is explained on the last page of this section.

Remember: All pregnancies have a background risk of 3% or more for a serious birth defect, even when mom doesn't take a drug of any kind. If you are pregnant or planning a pregnancy, always let your healthcare provider know before taking any drug, prescription or non-prescription, or herbal remedy.

Diabetic Tussin® Night Time Formula Cold, Flu Relief

Active Ingredient:	Pregnancy Risk Category:
Acetaminophen	B
Dextromethorphan Hbr	C
Diphenhydramine	B

Helpful Hints and Reminders: Each pregnancy risk category (**A**, **B**, **C**, **D**, or **X**) is explained on the last page of this section.

Remember: All pregnancies have a background risk of 3% or more for a serious birth defect, even when mom doesn't take a drug of any kind. If you are pregnant or planning a pregnancy, always let your healthcare provider know before taking any drug, prescription or non-prescription, or herbal remedy.

Dimetapp® Cold & Allergy Chewable Tablets

Active Ingredient:	Pregnancy Risk Category:
Brompheniramine maleate	C
Phenylephrine Hcl	C

Helpful Hints and Reminders: Each pregnancy risk category (**A**, **B**, **C**, **D**, or **X**) is explained on the last page of this section.

Remember: All pregnancies have a background risk of 3% or more for a serious birth defect, even when mom doesn't take a drug of any kind. If you are pregnant or planning a pregnancy, always let your healthcare provider know before taking any drug, prescription or non-prescription, or herbal remedy.

Dimetapp® Cold & Allergy Liquid

Active Ingredient:	Pregnancy Risk Category:
Brompheniramine maleate	C
Phenylephrine Hcl	C

Helpful Hints and Reminders: Each pregnancy risk category (**A**, **B**, **C**, **D**, or **X**) is explained on the last page of this section.

Remember: All pregnancies have a background risk of 3% or more for a serious birth defect, even when mom doesn't take a drug of any kind. If you are pregnant or planning a pregnancy, always let your healthcare provider know before taking any drug, prescription or non-prescription, or herbal remedy.

Dimetapp® Cold & Cough

Active Ingredient:	Pregnancy Risk Category:
Brompheniramine maleate	C
Phenylephrine Hcl	C
Dextromethorphan	C

Helpful Hints and Reminders: Each pregnancy risk category (**A**, **B**, **C**, **D**, or **X**) is explained on the last page of this section.

Remember: All pregnancies have a background risk of 3% or more for a serious birth defect, even when mom doesn't take a drug of any kind. If you are pregnant or planning a pregnancy, always let your healthcare provider know before taking any drug, prescription or non-prescription, or herbal remedy.

Dimetapp® Long Acting Cough Plus Cold

Active Ingredient:	Pregnancy Risk Category:
Dextromethorphan	C
Chlorpheniramine maleate	B

Helpful Hints and Reminders: Each pregnancy risk category (**A**, **B**, **C**, **D**, or **X**) is explained on the last page of this section.

Remember: All pregnancies have a background risk of 3% or more for a serious birth defect, even when mom doesn't take a drug of any kind. If you are pregnant or planning a pregnancy, always let your healthcare provider know before taking any drug, prescription or non-prescription, or herbal remedy.

Dimetapp® Nighttime Cold & Congestion

Active Ingredient:	Pregnancy Risk Category:
Phenylephrine Hcl	C
Diphenhydramine Hcl	B

Helpful Hints and Reminders: Each pregnancy risk category (**A**, **B**, **C**, **D**, or **X**) is explained on the last page of this section.

Remember: All pregnancies have a background risk of 3% or more for a serious birth defect, even when mom doesn't take a drug of any kind. If you are pregnant or planning a pregnancy, always let your healthcare provider know before taking any drug, prescription or non-prescription, or herbal remedy.

Dristan® Cold Multi-Symptom Nasal Decongestant Coated Tablets

Active Ingredient:	Pregnancy Risk Category:
Acetaminophen	B
Phenylephrine Hcl	C
Chlorpheniramine maleate	B

Helpful Hints and Reminders: Each pregnancy risk category (**A**, **B**, **C**, **D**, or **X**) is explained on the last page of this section.

Remember: All pregnancies have a background risk of 3% or more for a serious birth defect, even when mom doesn't take a drug of any kind. If you are pregnant or planning a pregnancy, always let your healthcare provider know before taking any drug, prescription or non-prescription, or herbal remedy.

Equate® Antihistabs Cold & Allergy Relief Tablets

Active Ingredient:	Pregnancy Risk Category:
Chlorpheniramine maleate	B
Phenylephrine Hcl	C

Helpful Hints and Reminders: Each pregnancy risk category (**A**, **B**, **C**, **D**, or **X**) is explained on the last page of this section.

Remember: All pregnancies have a background risk of 3% or more for a serious birth defect, even when mom doesn't take a drug of any kind. If you are pregnant or planning a pregnancy, always let your healthcare provider know before taking any drug, prescription or non-prescription, or herbal remedy.

Equate® Chest Congestion Tussin

Active Ingredient:	Pregnancy Risk Category:
Guaifenesin	C

Helpful Hints and Reminders: Each pregnancy risk category (**A**, **B**, **C**, **D**, or **X**) is explained on the last page of this section.

Remember: All pregnancies have a background risk of 3% or more for a serious birth defect, even when mom doesn't take a drug of any kind. If you are pregnant or planning a pregnancy, always let your healthcare provider know before taking any drug, prescription or non-prescription, or herbal remedy.

Equate® Cold Head Congestion Severe Pain Reliever Caplets

Active Ingredient:	Pregnancy Risk Category:
Acetaminophen	B
Dextromethorphan Hbr	C

(*continued*)

Phenylephrine Hcl	C
Guaifenesin	C

Helpful Hints and Reminders: Each pregnancy risk category (**A**, **B**, **C**, **D**, or **X**) is explained on the last page of this section.

Remember: All pregnancies have a background risk of 3% or more for a serious birth defect, even when mom doesn't take a drug of any kind. If you are pregnant or planning a pregnancy, always let your healthcare provider know before taking any drug, prescription or non-prescription, or herbal remedy.

Equate® Cold Multi-Symptom Daytime/Nighttime Value Pack Pain Reliever/Fever Reducer 2 pack

Active Ingredient:	Pregnancy Risk Category:
Daytime:	
Acetaminophen	B
Dextromethorphan Hbr	C
Phenylephrine Hcl	C
Nighttime:	
Acetaminophen	B
Dextromethorphan Hbr	C
Phenylephrine Hcl	C
Chlorpheniramine maleate	B

Helpful Hints and Reminders: Each pregnancy risk category (**A**, **B**, **C**, **D**, or **X**) is explained on the last page of this section.

Remember: All pregnancies have a background risk of 3% or more for a serious birth defect, even when mom doesn't take a drug of any kind. If you are pregnant or planning a pregnancy, always let your healthcare provider know before taking any drug, prescription or non-prescription, or herbal remedy.

Equate® Nite Time Cherry Flavor Multi-Symptom Cold/Flu Relief Liquid

Active Ingredient:	Pregnancy Risk Category:
Acetaminophen	B
Dextromethorphan Hbr	C
Doxylamine succinate	A

Helpful Hints and Reminders: Each pregnancy risk category (**A**, **B**, **C**, **D**, or **X**) is explained on the last page of this section.

Remember: All pregnancies have a background risk of 3% or more for a serious birth defect, even when mom doesn't take a drug of any kind. If you are pregnant or planning a pregnancy, always let your healthcare provider know before taking any drug, prescription or non-prescription, or herbal remedy.

Equate® Non-Drowsy Day Time Cold & Flu Multi-Symptom Relief Liquid

Active Ingredient:	Pregnancy Risk Category:
Acetaminophen	B
Dextromethorphan Hbr	C
Phenylephrine Hcl	C

Helpful Hints and Reminders: Each pregnancy risk category (**A**, **B**, **C**, **D**, or **X**) is explained on the last page of this section.

Remember: All pregnancies have a background risk of 3% or more for a serious birth defect, even when mom doesn't take a drug of any kind. If you are pregnant or planning a pregnancy, always let your healthcare provider know before taking any drug, prescription or non-prescription, or herbal remedy.

Equate® Tussin CF Cough & Cold Non-Drowsy

Active Ingredient:	Pregnancy Risk Category:
Dextromethorphan Hbr	C
Phenylephrine Hcl	C
Guaifenesin	C

Helpful Hints and Reminders: Each pregnancy risk category (**A**, **B**, **C**, **D**, or **X**) is explained on the last page of this section.

Remember: All pregnancies have a background risk of 3% or more for a serious birth defect, even when mom doesn't take a drug of any kind. If you are pregnant or planning a pregnancy, always let your healthcare provider know before taking any drug, prescription or non-prescription, or herbal remedy.

Equate® Tussin DM Cough Non-Drowsy Cough Suppressant/Expectorant

Active Ingredient:	Pregnancy Risk Category:
Dextromethorphan Hbr	C
Guaifenesin	C

Helpful Hints and Reminders: Each pregnancy risk category (**A**, **B**, **C**, **D**, or **X**) is explained on the last page of this section.

Remember: All pregnancies have a background risk of 3% or more for a serious birth defect, even when mom doesn't take a drug of any kind. If you are pregnant or planning a pregnancy, always let your healthcare provider know before taking any drug, prescription or non-prescription, or herbal remedy.

Father John's Medicine® Cough Suppressant

Active Ingredient:	Pregnancy Risk Category:
Dextromethorphan Hbr	C

Helpful Hints and Reminders: Each pregnancy risk category (**A**, **B**, **C**, **D**, or **X**) is explained on the last page of this section.

Remember: All pregnancies have a background risk of 3% or more for a serious birth defect, even when mom doesn't take a drug of any kind. If you are pregnant or planning a pregnancy, always let your healthcare provider know before taking any drug, prescription or non-prescription, or herbal remedy.

Mucinex®

Active Ingredient:	Pregnancy Risk Category:
Guaifenesin	C

Helpful Hints and Reminders: Each pregnancy risk category (**A**, **B**, **C**, **D**, or **X**) is explained on the last page of this section.

Remember: All pregnancies have a background risk of 3% or more for a serious birth defect, even when mom doesn't take a drug of any kind. If you are pregnant or planning a pregnancy, always let your healthcare provider know before taking any drug, prescription or non-prescription, or herbal remedy.

Mucinex® Cough Mini-Melts™

Active Ingredient:	Pregnancy Risk Category:
Dextromethorphan	C
Guaifenesin	C

Helpful Hints and Reminders: Each pregnancy risk category (**A**, **B**, **C**, **D**, or **X**) is explained on the last page of this section.

Remember: All pregnancies have a background risk of 3% or more for a serious birth defect, even when mom doesn't take a drug of any kind. If you are pregnant or planning a pregnancy, always let your healthcare provider know before taking any drug, prescription or non-prescription, or herbal remedy.

Mucinex® D

Active Ingredient:	Pregnancy Risk Category:
Guaifenesin	C
Pseudoephedrine Hcl	C

Helpful Hints and Reminders: Each pregnancy risk category (**A**, **B**, **C**, **D**, or **X**) is explained on the last page of this section.

Remember: All pregnancies have a background risk of 3% or more for a serious birth defect, even when mom doesn't take a drug of any kind. If you are pregnant or planning a pregnancy, always let your healthcare provider know before taking any drug, prescription or non-prescription, or herbal remedy.

Mucinex® D Maximum Strength

Active Ingredient:	Pregnancy Risk Category:
Guaifenesin	C
Pseudoephedrine Hcl	C

Helpful Hints and Reminders: Each pregnancy risk category (**A**, **B**, **C**, **D**, or **X**) is explained on the last page of this section.

Remember: All pregnancies have a background risk of 3% or more for a serious birth defect, even when mom doesn't take a drug of any kind. If you are pregnant or planning a pregnancy, always let your healthcare provider know before taking any drug, prescription or non-prescription, or herbal remedy.

Mucinex® DM

Active Ingredient:	Pregnancy Risk Category:
Dextromethorphan	C
Guaifenesin	C

Helpful Hints and Reminders: Each pregnancy risk category (**A**, **B**, **C**, **D**, or **X**) is explained on the last page of this section.

Remember: All pregnancies have a background risk of 3% or more for a serious birth defect, even when mom doesn't take a drug of any kind. If you are pregnant or planning a pregnancy, always let your healthcare provider know before taking any drug, prescription or non-prescription, or herbal remedy.

Mucinex® DM Maximum Strength

Active Ingredient:	Pregnancy Risk Category:
Dextromethorphan	C
Guaifenesin	C

Helpful Hints and Reminders: Each pregnancy risk category (**A**, **B**, **C**, **D**, or **X**) is explained on the last page of this section.

Remember: All pregnancies have a background risk of 3% or more for a serious birth defect, even when mom doesn't take a drug of any kind. If you are pregnant or planning a pregnancy, always let your healthcare provider know before taking any drug, prescription or non-prescription, or herbal remedy.

Mucinex® Mini-Melts™

Active Ingredient:	Pregnancy Risk Category:
Guaifenesin	C

Helpful Hints and Reminders: Each pregnancy risk category (**A**, **B**, **C**, **D**, or **X**) is explained on the last page of this section.

Remember: All pregnancies have a background risk of 3% or more for a serious birth defect, even when mom doesn't take a drug of any kind. If you are pregnant or planning a pregnancy, always let your healthcare provider know before taking any drug, prescription or non-prescription, or herbal remedy.

NyQuil® Cold & Flu Relief LiquiCaps

Active Ingredient:	Pregnancy Risk Category:
Acetaminophen	B
Doxylamine succinate	A
Dextromethorphan Hbr	C

Helpful Hints and Reminders: Each pregnancy risk category (**A**, **B**, **C**, **D**, or **X**) is explained on the last page of this section.

Remember: All pregnancies have a background risk of 3% or more for a serious birth defect, even when mom doesn't take a drug of any kind. If you are pregnant or planning a pregnancy, always let your healthcare provider know before taking any drug, prescription or non-prescription, or herbal remedy.

NyQuil® Cold & Flu Relief Liquid

Active Ingredient:	Pregnancy Risk Category:
Acetaminophen	B
Doxylamine succinate	A
Dextromethorphan Hbr	C

Helpful Hints and Reminders: Each pregnancy risk category (**A**, **B**, **C**, **D**, or **X**) is explained on the last page of this section.

Remember: All pregnancies have a background risk of 3% or more for a serious birth defect, even when mom doesn't take a drug of any kind. If you are pregnant or planning a pregnancy, always let your healthcare provider know before taking any drug, prescription or non-prescription, or herbal remedy.

NyQuil® Cold & Flu Symptom Relief Plus Vitamin C

Active Ingredient:	Pregnancy Risk Category:
Acetaminophen	**B**
Doxylamine succinate	**A**
Dextromethorphan Hbr	**C**

Helpful Hints and Reminders: Each pregnancy risk category (**A**, **B**, **C**, **D**, or **X**) is explained on the last page of this section.

Remember: All pregnancies have a background risk of 3% or more for a serious birth defect, even when mom doesn't take a drug of any kind. If you are pregnant or planning a pregnancy, always let your healthcare provider know before taking any drug, prescription or non-prescription, or herbal remedy.

NyQuil® Cough

Active Ingredient:	Pregnancy Risk Category:
Doxylamine succinate	**A**
Dextromethorphan Hbr	**C**

Helpful Hints and Reminders: Each pregnancy risk category (**A**, **B**, **C**, **D**, or **X**) is explained on the last page of this section.

Remember: All pregnancies have a background risk of 3% or more for a serious birth defect, even when mom doesn't take a drug of any kind. If you are pregnant or planning a pregnancy, always let your healthcare provider know before taking any drug, prescription or non-prescription, or herbal remedy.

Rite Aid® Mucus Relief Chest Immediate-Release Expectorant Tablets

Active Ingredient:	Pregnancy Risk Category:
Guaifenesin	**C**

Helpful Hints and Reminders: Each pregnancy risk category (**A**, **B**, **C**, **D**, or **X**) is explained on the last page of this section.

Remember: All pregnancies have a background risk of 3% or more for a serious birth defect, even when mom doesn't take a drug of any kind. If you are pregnant or planning a pregnancy, always let your healthcare provider know before taking any drug, prescription or non-prescription, or herbal remedy.

Rite Aid® Mucus Relief Sinus Expectorant/Decongestant

Active Ingredient:	Pregnancy Risk Category:
Guaifenesin	C
Phenylephrine Hcl	C

Helpful Hints and Reminders: Each pregnancy risk category (**A**, **B**, **C**, **D**, or **X**) is explained on the last page of this section.

Remember: All pregnancies have a background risk of 3% or more for a serious birth defect, even when mom doesn't take a drug of any kind. If you are pregnant or planning a pregnancy, always let your healthcare provider know before taking any drug, prescription or non-prescription, or herbal remedy.

Rite Aid® Multi-Symptom Nite Time Cold/Flu Formula

Active Ingredient:	Pregnancy Risk Category:
Acetaminophen	B
Dextromethorphan Hbr	C
Doxylamine succinate	A

Helpful Hints and Reminders: Each pregnancy risk category (**A**, **B**, **C**, **D**, or **X**) is explained on the last page of this section.

Remember: All pregnancies have a background risk of 3% or more for a serious birth defect, even when mom doesn't take a drug of any kind.

If you are pregnant or planning a pregnancy, always let your healthcare provider know before taking any drug, prescription or non-prescription, or herbal remedy.

Rite Aid® Nose Drops

Active Ingredient:	Pregnancy Risk Category:
Phenylephrine Hcl	C

Helpful Hints and Reminders: Each pregnancy risk category (**A**, **B**, **C**, **D**, or **X**) is explained on the last page of this section.

Remember: All pregnancies have a background risk of 3% or more for a serious birth defect, even when mom doesn't take a drug of any kind. If you are pregnant or planning a pregnancy, always let your healthcare provider know before taking any drug, prescription or non-prescription, or herbal remedy.

Rite Aid® Tussin Cough Suppressant Non-Drowsy

Active Ingredient:	Pregnancy Risk Category:
Dextromethorphan Hbr	C

Helpful Hints and Reminders: Each pregnancy risk category (**A**, **B**, **C**, **D**, or **X**) is explained on the last page of this section.

Remember: All pregnancies have a background risk of 3% or more for a serious birth defect, even when mom doesn't take a drug of any kind. If you are pregnant or planning a pregnancy, always let your healthcare provider know before taking any drug, prescription or non-prescription, or herbal remedy.

Robitussin® Cough & Cold CF Liquid

Active Ingredient:	Pregnancy Risk Category:
Dextromethorphan Hbr	C
Phenylephrine Hcl	C
Guaifenesin	C

Helpful Hints and Reminders: Each pregnancy risk category (**A**, **B**, **C**, **D**, or **X**) is explained on the last page of this section.

Remember: All pregnancies have a background risk of 3% or more for a serious birth defect, even when mom doesn't take a drug of any kind. If you are pregnant or planning a pregnancy, always let your healthcare provider know before taking any drug, prescription or non-prescription, or herbal remedy.

Robitussin® Cough & Cold Long Acting

Active Ingredient:	Pregnancy Risk Category:
Dextromethorphan Hbr	C
Chlorpheniramine maleate	B

Helpful Hints and Reminders: Each pregnancy risk category (**A**, **B**, **C**, **D**, or **X**) is explained on the last page of this section.

Remember: All pregnancies have a background risk of 3% or more for a serious birth defect, even when mom doesn't take a drug of any kind. If you are pregnant or planning a pregnancy, always let your healthcare provider know before taking any drug, prescription or non-prescription, or herbal remedy.

Robitussin® Cough & Congestion

Active Ingredient:	Pregnancy Risk Category:
Dextromethorphan Hbr	C
Guaifenesin	C

Helpful Hints and Reminders: Each pregnancy risk category (**A**, **B**, **C**, **D**, or **X**) is explained on the last page of this section.

Remember: All pregnancies have a background risk of 3% or more for a serious birth defect, even when mom doesn't take a drug of any kind. If you are pregnant or planning a pregnancy, always let your healthcare provider know before taking any drug, prescription or non-prescription, or herbal remedy.

Robitussin® Cough DM; Robitussin Sugar Free Cough

Active Ingredient:	Pregnancy Risk Category:
Dextromethorphan Hbr	C
Guaifenesin	C

Helpful Hints and Reminders: Each pregnancy risk category (**A**, **B**, **C**, **D**, or **X**) is explained on the last page of this section.

Remember: All pregnancies have a background risk of 3% or more for a serious birth defect, even when mom doesn't take a drug of any kind. If you are pregnant or planning a pregnancy, always let your healthcare provider know before taking any drug, prescription or non-prescription, or herbal remedy.

Robitussin® Cough Gels

Active Ingredient:	Pregnancy Risk Category:
Dextromethorphan Hbr	C

Helpful Hints and Reminders: Each pregnancy risk category (**A**, **B**, **C**, **D**, or **X**) is explained on the last page of this section.

Remember: All pregnancies have a background risk of 3% or more for a serious birth defect, even when mom doesn't take a drug of any kind. If you are pregnant or planning a pregnancy, always let your healthcare provider know before taking any drug, prescription or non-prescription, or herbal remedy.

Robitussin® Cough Long Acting

Active Ingredient:	Pregnancy Risk Category:
Dextromethorphan Hbr	C

Helpful Hints and Reminders: Each pregnancy risk category (**A**, **B**, **C**, **D**, or **X**) is explained on the last page of this section.

Remember: All pregnancies have a background risk of 3% or more for a serious birth defect, even when mom doesn't take a drug of any kind. If you are pregnant or planning a pregnancy, always let your healthcare provider know before taking any drug, prescription or non-prescription, or herbal remedy.

Robitussin® Head & Chest Congestion PE

Active Ingredient:	Pregnancy Risk Category:
Guaifenesin	C
Phenylephrine Hcl	C

Helpful Hints and Reminders: Each pregnancy risk category (**A**, **B**, **C**, **D**, or **X**) is explained on the last page of this section.

Remember: All pregnancies have a background risk of 3% or more for a serious birth defect, even when mom doesn't take a drug of any kind. If you are pregnant or planning a pregnancy, always let your healthcare provider know before taking any drug, prescription or non-prescription, or herbal remedy.

Robitussin® Nighttime Cough & Cold

Active Ingredient:	Pregnancy Risk Category:
Phenylephrine Hcl	C
Diphenhydramine Hcl	B

Helpful Hints and Reminders: Each pregnancy risk category (**A**, **B**, **C**, **D**, or **X**) is explained on the last page of this section.

Remember: All pregnancies have a background risk of 3% or more for a serious birth defect, even when mom doesn't take a drug of any kind. If you are pregnant or planning a pregnancy, always let your healthcare provider know before taking any drug, prescription or non-prescription, or herbal remedy.

Sudafed OM® Sinus Cold Spray

Active Ingredient:	Pregnancy Risk Category:
Oxymetazoline Hcl	C

Helpful Hints and Reminders: Each pregnancy risk category (**A**, **B**, **C**, **D**, or **X**) is explained on the last page of this section.

Remember: All pregnancies have a background risk of 3% or more for a serious birth defect, even when mom doesn't take a drug of any kind. If you are pregnant or planning a pregnancy, always let your healthcare provider know before taking any drug, prescription or non-prescription, or herbal remedy.

Sudafed OM® Sinus Congestion Spray

Active Ingredient:	Pregnancy Risk Category:
Oxymetazoline Hcl	C

Helpful Hints and Reminders: Each pregnancy risk category (**A**, **B**, **C**, **D**, or **X**) is explained on the last page of this section.

Remember: All pregnancies have a background risk of 3% or more for a serious birth defect, even when mom doesn't take a drug of any kind. If you are pregnant or planning a pregnancy, always let your healthcare provider know before taking any drug, prescription or non-prescription, or herbal remedy.

Sudafed PE® Cold and Cough Caplets

Active Ingredient:	Pregnancy Risk Category:
Acetaminophen	B
Phenylephrine Hcl	C
Dextromethorphan Hbr	C
Guaifenesin	C

Helpful Hints and Reminders: Each pregnancy risk category (**A**, **B**, **C**, **D**, or **X**) is explained on the last page of this section.

Remember: All pregnancies have a background risk of 3% or more for a serious birth defect, even when mom doesn't take a drug of any kind. If you are pregnant or planning a pregnancy, always let your healthcare provider know before taking any drug, prescription or non-prescription, or herbal remedy.

Sudafed PE® Day & Night Nasal Decongestant Tablets

Active Ingredient:	Pregnancy Risk Category:
Nighttime:	
Acetaminophen	B
Diphenhydramine Hcl	B
Phenylephrine Hcl	C
Daytime:	
Acetaminophen	B
Phenylephrine Hcl	C
Guaifenesin	C
Dextromethorphan Hbr	C

Helpful Hints and Reminders: Each pregnancy risk category (**A**, **B**, **C**, **D**, or **X**) is explained on the last page of this section.

Remember: All pregnancies have a background risk of 3% or more for a serious birth defect, even when mom doesn't take a drug of any kind.

If you are pregnant or planning a pregnancy, always let your healthcare provider know before taking any drug, prescription or non-prescription, or herbal remedy.

Sudafed PE® Nighttime Cold Caplets

Active Ingredient:	Pregnancy Risk Category:
Acetaminophen	B
Diphenhydramine Hcl	B
Phenylephrine Hcl	C

Helpful Hints and Reminders: Each pregnancy risk category (**A**, **B**, **C**, **D**, or **X**) is explained on the last page of this section.

Remember: All pregnancies have a background risk of 3% or more for a serious birth defect, even when mom doesn't take a drug of any kind. If you are pregnant or planning a pregnancy, always let your healthcare provider know before taking any drug, prescription or non-prescription, or herbal remedy.

Sudafed PE® Severe Cold Formula Caplets

Active Ingredient:	Pregnancy Risk Category:
Acetaminophen	B
Diphenhydramine Hcl	B
Phenylephrine Hcl	C

Helpful Hints and Reminders: Each pregnancy risk category (**A**, **B**, **C**, **D**, or **X**) is explained on the last page of this section.

Remember: All pregnancies have a background risk of 3% or more for a serious birth defect, even when mom doesn't take a drug of any kind. If you are pregnant or planning a pregnancy, always let your healthcare provider know before taking any drug, prescription or non-prescription, or herbal remedy.

Target® Cold PE Daytime Caplets

Active Ingredient:	Pregnancy Risk Category:
Acetaminophen	B
Phenylephrine Hcl	C
Dextromethorphan Hbr	C

Helpful Hints and Reminders: Each pregnancy risk category (**A**, **B**, **C**, **D**, or **X**) is explained on the last page of this section.

Remember: All pregnancies have a background risk of 3% or more for a serious birth defect, even when mom doesn't take a drug of any kind. If you are pregnant or planning a pregnancy, always let your healthcare provider know before taking any drug, prescription or non-prescription, or herbal remedy.

Target® Cough Relief DM Liquid

Active Ingredient:	Pregnancy Risk Category:
Dextromethorphan Hbr	C
Guaifenesin	C

Helpful Hints and Reminders: Each pregnancy risk category (**A**, **B**, **C**, **D**, or **X**) is explained on the last page of this section.

Remember: All pregnancies have a background risk of 3% or more for a serious birth defect, even when mom doesn't take a drug of any kind. If you are pregnant or planning a pregnancy, always let your healthcare provider know before taking any drug, prescription or non-prescription, or herbal remedy.

Target® Day/Night Cold/Flu Relief Softgels

Active Ingredient:	Pregnancy Risk Category:
Nighttime:	
Acetaminophen	B
Dextromethorphan	C
Doxylamine succinate	A
Daytime:	
Acetaminophen	B
Phenylephrine Hcl	C
Dextromethorphan Hbr	C

Helpful Hints and Reminders: Each pregnancy risk category (**A**, **B**, **C**, **D**, or **X**) is explained on the last page of this section.

Remember: All pregnancies have a background risk of 3% or more for a serious birth defect, even when mom doesn't take a drug of any kind. If you are pregnant or planning a pregnancy, always let your healthcare provider know before taking any drug, prescription or non-prescription, or herbal remedy.

Target® Maximum Strength Nasal Decongestant PE Tablets

Active Ingredient:	Pregnancy Risk Category:
Phenylephrine Hcl	C

Helpful Hints and Reminders: Each pregnancy risk category (**A**, **B**, **C**, **D**, or **X**) is explained on the last page of this section.

Remember: All pregnancies have a background risk of 3% or more for a serious birth defect, even when mom doesn't take a drug of any kind. If you are pregnant or planning a pregnancy, always let your healthcare provider know before taking any drug, prescription or non-prescription, or herbal remedy.

Target® Multi-Symptom Day/Night Combo Cold Relief Caplets

Active Ingredient:	Pregnancy Risk Category:
Nighttime:	
Acetaminophen	B
Dextromethorphan	C
Phenylephrine Hcl	C
Chlorpheniramine maleate	B
Daytime:	
Acetaminophen	B
Phenylephrine Hcl	C
Dextromethorphan Hbr	C

Helpful Hints and Reminders: Each pregnancy risk category (**A**, **B**, **C**, **D**, or **X**) is explained on the last page of this section.

Remember: All pregnancies have a background risk of 3% or more for a serious birth defect, even when mom doesn't take a drug of any kind. If you are pregnant or planning a pregnancy, always let your healthcare provider know before taking any drug, prescription or non-prescription, or herbal remedy.

Target® Multi-Symptom Daytime Cold & Flu Softgels

Active Ingredient:	Pregnancy Risk Category:
Acetaminophen	B
Phenylephrine Hcl	C
Dextromethorphan Hbr	C

Helpful Hints and Reminders: Each pregnancy risk category (**A**, **B**, **C**, **D**, or **X**) is explained on the last page of this section.

Remember: All pregnancies have a background risk of 3% or more for a serious birth defect, even when mom doesn't take a drug of any kind.

If you are pregnant or planning a pregnancy, always let your healthcare provider know before taking any drug, prescription or non-prescription, or herbal remedy.

Target® Multi-Symptom Nighttime Cold/Flu Relief Liquid

Active Ingredient:	Pregnancy Risk Category:
Acetaminophen	B
Dextromethorphan Hbr	C
Doxylamine succinate	A

Helpful Hints and Reminders: Each pregnancy risk category (**A**, **B**, **C**, **D**, or **X**) is explained on the last page of this section.

Remember: All pregnancies have a background risk of 3% or more for a serious birth defect, even when mom doesn't take a drug of any kind. If you are pregnant or planning a pregnancy, always let your healthcare provider know before taking any drug, prescription or non-prescription, or herbal remedy.

Target® Nighttime Cold/Flu Relief

Active Ingredient:	Pregnancy Risk Category:
Acetaminophen	B
Dextromethorphan Hbr	C
Doxylamine succinate	A

Helpful Hints and Reminders: Each pregnancy risk category (**A**, **B**, **C**, **D**, or **X**) is explained on the last page of this section.

Remember: All pregnancies have a background risk of 3% or more for a serious birth defect, even when mom doesn't take a drug of any kind. If you are pregnant or planning a pregnancy, always let your healthcare provider know before taking any drug, prescription or non-prescription, or herbal remedy.

Theraflu® Caplets Daytime Severe Cold

Active Ingredient:	Pregnancy Risk Category:
Acetaminophen	B
Phenylephrine Hcl	C
Dextromethorphan Hbr	C

Helpful Hints and Reminders: Each pregnancy risk category (**A**, **B**, **C**, **D**, or **X**) is explained on the last page of this section.

Remember: All pregnancies have a background risk of 3% or more for a serious birth defect, even when mom doesn't take a drug of any kind. If you are pregnant or planning a pregnancy, always let your healthcare provider know before taking any drug, prescription or non-prescription, or herbal remedy.

Theraflu® Caplets Nighttime Severe Cold

Active Ingredient:	Pregnancy Risk Category:
Acetaminophen	B
Phenylephrine Hcl	C
Dextromethorphan Hbr	C
Chlorpheniramine maleate	B

Helpful Hints and Reminders: Each pregnancy risk category (**A**, **B**, **C**, **D**, or **X**) is explained on the last page of this section.

Remember: All pregnancies have a background risk of 3% or more for a serious birth defect, even when mom doesn't take a drug of any kind. If you are pregnant or planning a pregnancy, always let your healthcare provider know before taking any drug, prescription or non-prescription, or herbal remedy.

Theraflu® Cold & Cough

Active Ingredient:	Pregnancy Risk Category:
Phenylephrine Hcl	C
Dextromethorphan Hbr	C
Pheniramine maleate	C

Helpful Hints and Reminders: Each pregnancy risk category (**A**, **B**, **C**, **D**, or **X**) is explained on the last page of this section.

Remember: All pregnancies have a background risk of 3% or more for a serious birth defect, even when mom doesn't take a drug of any kind. If you are pregnant or planning a pregnancy, always let your healthcare provider know before taking any drug, prescription or non-prescription, or herbal remedy.

Theraflu® Cold & Sore Throat

Active Ingredient:	Pregnancy Risk Category:
Acetaminophen	B
Pheniramine maleate	C
Phenylephrine Hcl	C

Helpful Hints and Reminders: Each pregnancy risk category (**A**, **B**, **C**, **D**, or **X**) is explained on the last page of this section.

Remember: All pregnancies have a background risk of 3% or more for a serious birth defect, even when mom doesn't take a drug of any kind. If you are pregnant or planning a pregnancy, always let your healthcare provider know before taking any drug, prescription or non-prescription, or herbal remedy.

Theraflu® Daytime Severe Cold

Active Ingredient:	Pregnancy Risk Category:
Acetaminophen	B
Phenylephrine Hcl	C

Theraflu® Flu & Sore Throat

Helpful Hints and Reminders: Each pregnancy risk category (**A**, **B**, **C**, **D**, or **X**) is explained on the last page of this section.

Remember: All pregnancies have a background risk of 3% or more for a serious birth defect, even when mom doesn't take a drug of any kind. If you are pregnant or planning a pregnancy, always let your healthcare provider know before taking any drug, prescription or non-prescription, or herbal remedy.

Theraflu® Flu & Chest Congestion

Active Ingredient:	Pregnancy Risk Category:
Acetaminophen	B
Guaifenesin	C

Helpful Hints and Reminders: Each pregnancy risk category (**A**, **B**, **C**, **D**, or **X**) is explained on the last page of this section.

Remember: All pregnancies have a background risk of 3% or more for a serious birth defect, even when mom doesn't take a drug of any kind. If you are pregnant or planning a pregnancy, always let your healthcare provider know before taking any drug, prescription or non-prescription, or herbal remedy.

Theraflu® Flu & Sore Throat

Active Ingredient:	Pregnancy Risk Category:
Acetaminophen	B
Pheniramine maleate	C
Phenylephrine Hcl	C

Helpful Hints and Reminders: Each pregnancy risk category (**A**, **B**, **C**, **D**, or **X**) is explained on the last page of this section.

Remember: All pregnancies have a background risk of 3% or more for a serious birth defect, even when mom doesn't take a drug of any kind. If you are pregnant or planning a pregnancy, always let your healthcare provider know before taking any drug, prescription or non-prescription, or herbal remedy.

Theraflu® Nighttime Severe Cold

Active Ingredient:	Pregnancy Risk Category:
Acetaminophen	B
Pheniramine maleate	C
Phenylephrine Hcl	C

Helpful Hints and Reminders: Each pregnancy risk category (**A**, **B**, **C**, **D**, or **X**) is explained on the last page of this section.

Remember: All pregnancies have a background risk of 3% or more for a serious birth defect, even when mom doesn't take a drug of any kind. If you are pregnant or planning a pregnancy, always let your healthcare provider know before taking any drug, prescription or non-prescription, or herbal remedy.

Theraflu® Thinstrips Daytime Cold & Cough

Active Ingredient:	Pregnancy Risk Category:
Phenylephrine Hcl	C
Dextromethorphan Hbr	C

Helpful Hints and Reminders: Each pregnancy risk category (**A**, **B**, **C**, **D**, or **X**) is explained on the last page of this section.

Remember: All pregnancies have a background risk of 3% or more for a serious birth defect, even when mom doesn't take a drug of any kind. If you are pregnant or planning a pregnancy, always let your healthcare provider know before taking any drug, prescription or non-prescription, or herbal remedy.

Theraflu® Thinstrips Nighttime Cold & Cough

Active Ingredient:	Pregnancy Risk Category:
Diphenhydramine Hcl	B
Phenylephrine Hcl	C

Helpful Hints and Reminders: Each pregnancy risk category (**A**, **B**, **C**, **D**, or **X**) is explained on the last page of this section.

Remember: All pregnancies have a background risk of 3% or more for a serious birth defect, even when mom doesn't take a drug of any kind. If you are pregnant or planning a pregnancy, always let your healthcare provider know before taking any drug, prescription or non-prescription, or herbal remedy.

Theraflu® Warming Relief Daytime Severe Cold

Active Ingredient:	Pregnancy Risk Category:
Acetaminophen	B
Phenylephrine Hcl	C
Dextromethorphan Hbr	C

Helpful Hints and Reminders: Each pregnancy risk category (**A**, **B**, **C**, **D**, or **X**) is explained on the last page of this section.

Remember: All pregnancies have a background risk of 3% or more for a serious birth defect, even when mom doesn't take a drug of any kind. If you are pregnant or planning a pregnancy, always let your healthcare provider know before taking any drug, prescription or non-prescription, or herbal remedy.

Theraflu® Warming Relief Nighttime Severe Cold

Active Ingredient:	Pregnancy Risk Category:
Diphenhydramine Hcl	B
Phenylephrine Hcl	C
Acetaminophen	B

Helpful Hints and Reminders: Each pregnancy risk category (**A**, **B**, **C**, **D**, or **X**) is explained on the last page of this section.

Remember: All pregnancies have a background risk of 3% or more for a serious birth defect, even when mom doesn't take a drug of any kind.

If you are pregnant or planning a pregnancy, always let your healthcare provider know before taking any drug, prescription or non-prescription, or herbal remedy.

Tylenol® Cold Head Congestion Day/Night Pack

Active Ingredient:	Pregnancy Risk Category:
Daytime:	
Acetaminophen	B
Dextromethorphan Hbr	C
Phenylephrine Hcl	C
Nighttime:	
Acetaminophen	B
Dextromethorphan Hbr	C
Phenylephrine Hcl	C
Chlorpheniramine maleate	B

Helpful Hints and Reminders: Each pregnancy risk category (**A**, **B**, **C**, **D**, or **X**) is explained on the last page of this section.

Remember: All pregnancies have a background risk of 3% or more for a serious birth defect, even when mom doesn't take a drug of any kind. If you are pregnant or planning a pregnancy, always let your healthcare provider know before taking any drug, prescription or non-prescription, or herbal remedy.

Tylenol® Cold Head Congestion Daytime

Active Ingredient:	Pregnancy Risk Category:
Acetaminophen	B
Dextromethorphan Hbr	C
Phenylephrine Hcl	C

Helpful Hints and Reminders: Each pregnancy risk category (**A**, **B**, **C**, **D**, or **X**) is explained on the last page of this section.

Remember: All pregnancies have a background risk of 3% or more for a serious birth defect, even when mom doesn't take a drug of any kind. If you are pregnant or planning a pregnancy, always let your healthcare provider know before taking any drug, prescription or non-prescription, or herbal remedy.

Tylenol® Cold Head Congestion Nighttime

Active Ingredient:	Pregnancy Risk Category:
Acetaminophen	B
Dextromethorphan Hbr	C
Phenylephrine Hcl	C
Chlorpheniramine maleate	B

Helpful Hints and Reminders: Each pregnancy risk category (**A**, **B**, **C**, **D**, or **X**) is explained on the last page of this section.

Remember: All pregnancies have a background risk of 3% or more for a serious birth defect, even when mom doesn't take a drug of any kind. If you are pregnant or planning a pregnancy, always let your healthcare provider know before taking any drug, prescription or non-prescription, or herbal remedy.

Tylenol® Cold Head Congestion Severe

Active Ingredient:	Pregnancy Risk Category:
Acetaminophen	B
Dextromethorphan Hbr	C
Guaifenesin	C
Pseudoephedrine Hcl	C

Helpful Hints and Reminders: Each pregnancy risk category (**A**, **B**, **C**, **D**, or **X**) is explained on the last page of this section.

Remember: All pregnancies have a background risk of 3% or more for a serious birth defect, even when mom doesn't take a drug of any kind. If you are pregnant or planning a pregnancy, always let your healthcare provider know before taking any drug, prescription or non-prescription, or herbal remedy.

Tylenol® Cold Multi-Symptom Day/Night Pack

Active Ingredient:	Pregnancy Risk Category:
Daytime:	
Acetaminophen	B
Dextromethorphan Hbr	C
Phenylephrine Hcl	C
Nighttime:	
Acetaminophen	B
Dextromethorphan Hbr	C
Phenylephrine Hcl	C
Chlorpheniramine maleate	B

Helpful Hints and Reminders: Each pregnancy risk category (**A**, **B**, **C**, **D**, or **X**) is explained on the last page of this section.

Remember: All pregnancies have a background risk of 3% or more for a serious birth defect, even when mom doesn't take a drug of any kind. If you are pregnant or planning a pregnancy, always let your healthcare provider know before taking any drug, prescription or non-prescription, or herbal remedy.

Tylenol® Cold Multi-Symptom Daytime

Active Ingredient:	Pregnancy Risk Category:
Acetaminophen	B
Dextromethorphan Hbr	C
Phenylephrine Hcl	C

Tylenol® Cold Multi-Symptom Severe

Helpful Hints and Reminders: Each pregnancy risk category (**A**, **B**, **C**, **D**, or **X**) is explained on the last page of this section.

Remember: All pregnancies have a background risk of 3% or more for a serious birth defect, even when mom doesn't take a drug of any kind. If you are pregnant or planning a pregnancy, always let your healthcare provider know before taking any drug, prescription or non-prescription, or herbal remedy.

Tylenol® Cold Multi-Symptom Nighttime

Active Ingredient:	Pregnancy Risk Category:
Acetaminophen	B
Dextromethorphan Hbr	C
Phenylephrine Hcl	C
Chlorpheniramine maleate	B

Helpful Hints and Reminders: Each pregnancy risk category (**A**, **B**, **C**, **D**, or **X**) is explained on the last page of this section.

Remember: All pregnancies have a background risk of 3% or more for a serious birth defect, even when mom doesn't take a drug of any kind. If you are pregnant or planning a pregnancy, always let your healthcare provider know before taking any drug, prescription or non-prescription, or herbal remedy.

Tylenol® Cold Multi-Symptom Severe

Active Ingredient:	Pregnancy Risk Category:
Acetaminophen	B
Dextromethorphan Hbr	C
Phenylephrine Hcl	C
Guaifenesin	C

Helpful Hints and Reminders: Each pregnancy risk category (**A**, **B**, **C**, **D**, or **X**) is explained on the last page of this section.

Remember: All pregnancies have a background risk of 3% or more for a serious birth defect, even when mom doesn't take a drug of any kind. If you are pregnant or planning a pregnancy, always let your healthcare provider know before taking any drug, prescription or non-prescription, or herbal remedy.

Tylenol® Cold Severe Congestion Daytime

Active Ingredient:	Pregnancy Risk Category:
Acetaminophen	B
Dextromethorphan Hbr	C
Guaifenesin	C
Pseudoephedrine Hcl	C

Helpful Hints and Reminders: Each pregnancy risk category (**A**, **B**, **C**, **D**, or **X**) is explained on the last page of this section.

Remember: All pregnancies have a background risk of 3% or more for a serious birth defect, even when mom doesn't take a drug of any kind. If you are pregnant or planning a pregnancy, always let your healthcare provider know before taking any drug, prescription or non-prescription, or herbal remedy.

Up & Up™ Mucus Relief DM

Active Ingredient:	Pregnancy Risk Category:
Guaifenesin	C

Helpful Hints and Reminders: Each pregnancy risk category (**A**, **B**, **C**, **D**, or **X**) is explained on the last page of this section.

Remember: All pregnancies have a background risk of 3% or more for a serious birth defect, even when mom doesn't take a drug of any kind. If you are pregnant or planning a pregnancy, always let your healthcare provider know before taking any drug, prescription or non-prescription, or herbal remedy.

Vicks® Formula 44® Custom Care™ Chesty Cough

Active Ingredient:	Pregnancy Risk Category:
Dextromethorphan Hbr	C
Guaifenesin	C

Helpful Hints and Reminders: Each pregnancy risk category (**A**, **B**, **C**, **D**, or **X**) is explained on the last page of this section.

Remember: All pregnancies have a background risk of 3% or more for a serious birth defect, even when mom doesn't take a drug of any kind. If you are pregnant or planning a pregnancy, always let your healthcare provider know before taking any drug, prescription or non-prescription, or herbal remedy.

Vicks® Formula 44® Custom Care™ Congestion

Active Ingredient:	Pregnancy Risk Category:
Dextromethorphan Hbr	C
Phenylephrine Hcl	C

Helpful Hints and Reminders: Each pregnancy risk category (**A**, **B**, **C**, **D**, or **X**) is explained on the last page of this section.

Remember: All pregnancies have a background risk of 3% or more for a serious birth defect, even when mom doesn't take a drug of any kind. If you are pregnant or planning a pregnancy, always let your healthcare provider know before taking any drug, prescription or non-prescription, or herbal remedy.

Vicks® Formula 44® Custom Care™ Cough & Cold PM

Active Ingredient:	Pregnancy Risk Category:
Acetaminophen	B
Dextromethorphan	C
Chlorpheniramine maleate	B

Helpful Hints and Reminders: Each pregnancy risk category (**A**, **B**, **C**, **D**, or **X**) is explained on the last page of this section.

Remember: All pregnancies have a background risk of 3% or more for a serious birth defect, even when mom doesn't take a drug of any kind. If you are pregnant or planning a pregnancy, always let your healthcare provider know before taking any drug, prescription or non-prescription, or herbal remedy.

Vicks® Formula 44® Custom Care™ Dry Cough Suppressant

Active Ingredient:	Pregnancy Risk Category:
Dextromethorphan Hbr	C

Helpful Hints and Reminders: Each pregnancy risk category (**A**, **B**, **C**, **D**, or **X**) is explained on the last page of this section.

Remember: All pregnancies have a background risk of 3% or more for a serious birth defect, even when mom doesn't take a drug of any kind. If you are pregnant or planning a pregnancy, always let your healthcare provider know before taking any drug, prescription or non-prescription, or herbal remedy.

Vicks® Sinex® VapoSpray™ 4-Hour

Active Ingredient:	Pregnancy Risk Category:
Phenylephrine Hcl	C

Vicks® Sinex® VapoSpray™ Moisturizing

Helpful Hints and Reminders: Each pregnancy risk category (**A**, **B**, **C**, **D**, or **X**) is explained on the last page of this section.

Remember: All pregnancies have a background risk of 3% or more for a serious birth defect, even when mom doesn't take a drug of any kind. If you are pregnant or planning a pregnancy, always let your healthcare provider know before taking any drug, prescription or non-prescription, or herbal remedy.

Vicks® Sinex® VapoSpray™ 12-hour Decongestant Nasal Spray

Active Ingredient:	Pregnancy Risk Category:
Oxymetazoline Hcl	C

Helpful Hints and Reminders: Each pregnancy risk category (**A**, **B**, **C**, **D**, or **X**) is explained on the last page of this section.

Remember: All pregnancies have a background risk of 3% or more for a serious birth defect, even when mom doesn't take a drug of any kind. If you are pregnant or planning a pregnancy, always let your healthcare provider know before taking any drug, prescription or non-prescription, or herbal remedy.

Vicks® Sinex® VapoSpray™ Moisturizing 12-Hour Decongestant UltraFine Mist

Active Ingredient:	Pregnancy Risk Category:
Oxymetazoline Hcl	C

Helpful Hints and Reminders: Each pregnancy risk category (**A**, **B**, **C**, **D**, or **X**) is explained on the last page of this section.

Remember: All pregnancies have a background risk of 3% or more for a serious birth defect, even when mom doesn't take a drug of any kind. If you are pregnant or planning a pregnancy, always let your healthcare provider know before taking any drug, prescription or non-prescription, or herbal remedy.

Vicks® Sinex® VapoSpray™ 12-Hour Decongestant UltraFine Mist

Active Ingredient:	Pregnancy Risk Category:
Oxymetazoline Hcl	C

Helpful Hints and Reminders: Each pregnancy risk category (**A**, **B**, **C**, **D**, or **X**) is explained on the last page of this section.

Remember: All pregnancies have a background risk of 3% or more for a serious birth defect, even when mom doesn't take a drug of any kind. If you are pregnant or planning a pregnancy, always let your healthcare provider know before taking any drug, prescription or non-prescription, or herbal remedy.

Vicks® VapoSyrup™ Severe Congestion Head & Chest Congestion Relief

Active Ingredient:	Pregnancy Risk Category:
Guaifenesin	C
Phenylephrine Hcl	C

Helpful Hints and Reminders: Each pregnancy risk category (**A**, **B**, **C**, **D**, or **X**) is explained on the last page of this section.

Remember: All pregnancies have a background risk of 3% or more for a serious birth defect, even when mom doesn't take a drug of any kind. If you are pregnant or planning a pregnancy, always let your healthcare provider know before taking any drug, prescription or non-prescription, or herbal remedy.

XL-3® Cold Medicine Tablets

Active Ingredient:	Pregnancy Risk Category:
Acetaminophen	B
Chlorpheniramine maleate	B
Phenylephrine Hcl	C

Helpful Hints and Reminders: Each pregnancy risk category (**A**, **B**, **C**, **D**, or **X**) is explained on the last page of this section.

Remember: All pregnancies have a background risk of 3% or more for a serious birth defect, even when mom doesn't take a drug of any kind. If you are pregnant or planning a pregnancy, always let your healthcare provider know before taking any drug, prescription or non-prescription, or herbal remedy.

Zicam® Cough Max Cough Melts

Active Ingredient:	Pregnancy Risk Category:
Dextromethorphan Hbr	C

Helpful Hints and Reminders: Each pregnancy risk category (**A**, **B**, **C**, **D**, or **X**) is explained on the last page of this section.

Remember: All pregnancies have a background risk of 3% or more for a serious birth defect, even when mom doesn't take a drug of any kind. If you are pregnant or planning a pregnancy, always let your healthcare provider know before taking any drug, prescription or non-prescription, or herbal remedy.

Zicam® Cough Max Cough Spray

Active Ingredient:	Pregnancy Risk Category:
Dextromethorphan Hbr	C

Helpful Hints and Reminders: Each pregnancy risk category (**A**, **B**, **C**, **D**, or **X**) is explained on the last page of this section.

Remember: All pregnancies have a background risk of 3% or more for a serious birth defect, even when mom doesn't take a drug of any kind. If you are pregnant or planning a pregnancy, always let your healthcare provider know before taking any drug, prescription or non-prescription, or herbal remedy.

Zicam® Multi-Symptom Cold & Flu Daytime To Go

Active Ingredient:	Pregnancy Risk Category:
Acetaminophen	B
Dextromethorphan Hbr	C
Chlorpheniramine maleate	B
Phenylephrine Hcl	C

Helpful Hints and Reminders: Each pregnancy risk category (**A**, **B**, **C**, **D**, or **X**) is explained on the last page of this section.

Remember: All pregnancies have a background risk of 3% or more for a serious birth defect, even when mom doesn't take a drug of any kind. If you are pregnant or planning a pregnancy, always let your healthcare provider know before taking any drug, prescription or non-prescription, or herbal remedy.

Zicam® Multi-Symptom Cold & Flu Liquid Daytime

Active Ingredient:	Pregnancy Risk Category:
Acetaminophen	B
Dextromethorphan Hbr	C
Guaifenesin	C

Helpful Hints and Reminders: Each pregnancy risk category (**A**, **B**, **C**, **D**, or **X**) is explained on the last page of this section.

Remember: All pregnancies have a background risk of 3% or more for a serious birth defect, even when mom doesn't take a drug of any kind. If you are pregnant or planning a pregnancy, always let your healthcare provider know before taking any drug, prescription or non-prescription, or herbal remedy.

Zicam® Multi-Symptom Cold & Flu Nighttime To Go

Zicam® Multi-Symptom Cold & Flu Nighttime Liquid

Active Ingredient:	Pregnancy Risk Category:
Acetaminophen	**B**
Dextromethorphan Hbr	**C**
Doxylamine succinate	**A**

Helpful Hints and Reminders: Each pregnancy risk category (**A**, **B**, **C**, **D**, or **X**) is explained on the last page of this section.

Remember: All pregnancies have a background risk of 3% or more for a serious birth defect, even when mom doesn't take a drug of any kind. If you are pregnant or planning a pregnancy, always let your healthcare provider know before taking any drug, prescription or non-prescription, or herbal remedy.

Zicam® Multi-Symptom Cold & Flu Nighttime To Go

Active Ingredient:	Pregnancy Risk Category:
Acetaminophen	**B**
Dextromethorphan Hbr	**C**
Phenylephrine Hcl	**C**
Doxylamine succinate	**A**

Helpful Hints and Reminders: Each pregnancy risk category (**A**, **B**, **C**, **D**, or **X**) is explained on the last page of this section.

Remember: All pregnancies have a background risk of 3% or more for a serious birth defect, even when mom doesn't take a drug of any kind. If you are pregnant or planning a pregnancy, always let your healthcare provider know before taking any drug, prescription or non-prescription, or herbal remedy.

The FDA's Pregnancy Risk Categories: A, B, C, D, X

Adapted to the Active Ingredients in Nonprescription drugs

Category A: Controlled studies using the active ingredient in pregnant women have not shown harmful fetal effects throughout pregnancy, and the possibility of fetal harm seems remote. My comment: *Though apparently safe, these active ingredients should still only be used in pregnancy when clearly indicated.*

Category B: Either studies have shown no evidence of fetal harm when using the active ingredient in pregnant animals, but no controlled studies have been done in pregnant women, **or** studies have shown evidence of fetal harm when using the active ingredient in pregnant animals, but controlled studies in pregnant women have not shown evidence of fetal harm. My comment: *These active ingredients should only be used in pregnancy when clearly indicated.*

Category C: Either studies have shown evidence of fetal harm when using the active ingredient in pregnant animals, but no controlled studies have been done in pregnant women, **or** studies using the active ingredient in pregnant animals have not been done, and studies of pregnant women are insufficient to reach a conclusion. These active ingredients should only be used by a pregnant woman if the potential benefit justifies the potential risk of fetal harm, which, in many cases, is unknown. My comment: *It's impossible to calculate the potential risk of fetal harm when, in many cases, it's unknown. Thus, these active ingredients should only be used in pregnancy when clearly needed.*

Category D: Studies have shown evidence of fetal harm when using the active ingredient in pregnant women. However, the potential benefit of using the active ingredient in some life-threatening situations for

mom may outweigh the potential risk of fetal harm. For example, when mom requires cancer treatment or when she has a serious disease for which safer active ingredients cannot be used or are less effective. My comment: *These exceptional indications rarely occur when considering a nonprescription drug in pregnancy.*

Category X: My comment: *Because the risk of fetal harm is too high, no Category X active ingredients have been approved for use in nonprescription drugs.*

Active Ingredients Assigned Two Pregnancy Risk Categories: Some active ingredients have two pregnancy risk categories, depending on which trimester of pregnancy the active ingredient is used. For example, naproxen sodium, the active ingredient in Aleve, belongs to Category **B** when used in the first and second trimesters of pregnancy. If used in the third trimester, however, the active ingredient belongs to Category **D**. My comment: *This means naproxen sodium should not be used in the third trimester unless prescribed by a physician who has advised her patient of the risks involved.*

Section 3: Constipation

Alophen® Tablets

Active Ingredient:	Pregnancy Risk Category:
Bisacodyl	C

Helpful Hints and Reminders: Each pregnancy risk category (**A**, **B**, **C**, **D**, or **X**) is explained on the last page of this section.

Remember: All pregnancies have a background risk of 3% or more for a serious birth defect, even when mom doesn't take a drug of any kind. If you are pregnant or planning a pregnancy, always let your healthcare provider know before taking any drug, prescription or non-prescription, or herbal remedy.

• •

Carter's® Laxative Tablets

Active Ingredient:	Pregnancy Risk Category:
Bisacodyl	C

Helpful Hints and Reminders: Each pregnancy risk category (**A**, **B**, **C**, **D**, or **X**) is explained on the last page of this section.

Remember: All pregnancies have a background risk of 3% or more for a serious birth defect, even when mom doesn't take a drug of any kind. If you are pregnant or planning a pregnancy, always let your healthcare

provider know before taking any drug, prescription or non-prescription, or herbal remedy.

Colace® Stool Softener Capsules

Active Ingredient:	Pregnancy Risk Category:
Docusate sodium	C

Helpful Hints and Reminders: Each pregnancy risk category (**A**, **B**, **C**, **D**, or **X**) is explained on the last page of this section.

Remember: All pregnancies have a background risk of 3% or more for a serious birth defect, even when mom doesn't take a drug of any kind. If you are pregnant or planning a pregnancy, always let your healthcare provider know before taking any drug, prescription or non-prescription, or herbal remedy.

Colace® Stool Softener Liquid 1% Solution

Active Ingredient:	Pregnancy Risk Category:
Docusate sodium	C

Helpful Hints and Reminders: Each pregnancy risk category (**A**, **B**, **C**, **D**, or **X**) is explained on the last page of this section.

Remember: All pregnancies have a background risk of 3% or more for a serious birth defect, even when mom doesn't take a drug of any kind. If you are pregnant or planning a pregnancy, always let your healthcare provider know before taking any drug, prescription or non-prescription, or herbal remedy.

Colace® Stool Softener Syrup

Active Ingredient:	Pregnancy Risk Category:
Docusate sodium	C

Helpful Hints and Reminders: Each pregnancy risk category (**A**, **B**, **C**, **D**, or **X**) is explained on the last page of this section.

Remember: All pregnancies have a background risk of 3% or more for a serious birth defect, even when mom doesn't take a drug of any kind. If you are pregnant or planning a pregnancy, always let your healthcare provider know before taking any drug, prescription or non-prescription, or herbal remedy.

Colace® Glycerin Suppositories

Active Ingredient:	Pregnancy Risk Category:
Glycerin	C

Helpful Hints and Reminders: Each pregnancy risk category (**A**, **B**, **C**, **D**, or **X**) is explained on the last page of this section.

Remember: All pregnancies have a background risk of 3% or more for a serious birth defect, even when mom doesn't take a drug of any kind. If you are pregnant or planning a pregnancy, always let your healthcare provider know before taking any drug, prescription or non-prescription, or herbal remedy.

Correctol® Laxative Tablets

Active Ingredient:	Pregnancy Risk Category:
Bisacodyl	C

Helpful Hints and Reminders: Each pregnancy risk category (**A**, **B**, **C**, **D**, or **X**) is explained on the last page of this section.

Remember: All pregnancies have a background risk of 3% or more for a serious birth defect, even when mom doesn't take a drug of any kind. If you are pregnant or planning a pregnancy, always let your healthcare provider know before taking any drug, prescription or non-prescription, or herbal remedy.

CVS® Gentle Laxative Suppositories

Active Ingredient:	Pregnancy Risk Category:
Bisacodyl	C

Helpful Hints and Reminders: Each pregnancy risk category (**A**, **B**, **C**, **D**, or **X**) is explained on the last page of this section.

Remember: All pregnancies have a background risk of 3% or more for a serious birth defect, even when mom doesn't take a drug of any kind. If you are pregnant or planning a pregnancy, always let your healthcare provider know before taking any drug, prescription or non-prescription, or herbal remedy.

CVS® Gentle Laxative Tablets

Active Ingredient:	Pregnancy Risk Category:
Bisacodyl	C

Helpful Hints and Reminders: Each pregnancy risk category (**A**, **B**, **C**, **D**, or **X**) is explained on the last page of this section.

Remember: All pregnancies have a background risk of 3% or more for a serious birth defect, even when mom doesn't take a drug of any kind. If you are pregnant or planning a pregnancy, always let your healthcare provider know before taking any drug, prescription or non-prescription, or herbal remedy.

CVS® Stool Softener Capsules Original

Active Ingredient:	Pregnancy Risk Category:
Docusate sodium	C

Helpful Hints and Reminders: Each pregnancy risk category (**A**, **B**, **C**, **D**, or **X**) is explained on the last page of this section.

Remember: All pregnancies have a background risk of 3% or more for a serious birth defect, even when mom doesn't take a drug of any kind. If you are pregnant or planning a pregnancy, always let your healthcare

provider know before taking any drug, prescription or non-prescription, or herbal remedy.

CVS® Stool Softener Softgels

Active Ingredient:	Pregnancy Risk Category:
Docusate sodium	C

Helpful Hints and Reminders: Each pregnancy risk category (**A**, **B**, **C**, **D**, or **X**) is explained on the last page of this section.

Remember: All pregnancies have a background risk of 3% or more for a serious birth defect, even when mom doesn't take a drug of any kind. If you are pregnant or planning a pregnancy, always let your healthcare provider know before taking any drug, prescription or non-prescription, or herbal remedy.

Dulcolax® Balance

Active Ingredient:	Pregnancy Risk Category:
Polyethylene Glycol 3350	C

Helpful Hints and Reminders: Each pregnancy risk category (**A**, **B**, **C**, **D**, or **X**) is explained on the last page of this section.

Remember: All pregnancies have a background risk of 3% or more for a serious birth defect, even when mom doesn't take a drug of any kind. If you are pregnant or planning a pregnancy, always let your healthcare provider know before taking any drug, prescription or non-prescription, or herbal remedy.

Dulcolax® Laxative Suppositories

Active Ingredient:	Pregnancy Risk Category:
Bisacodyl	C

Helpful Hints and Reminders: Each pregnancy risk category (**A**, **B**, **C**, **D**, or **X**) is explained on the last page of this section.

Remember: All pregnancies have a background risk of 3% or more for a serious birth defect, even when mom doesn't take a drug of any kind. If you are pregnant or planning a pregnancy, always let your healthcare provider know before taking any drug, prescription or non-prescription, or herbal remedy.

Dulcolax® Laxative Tablets

Active Ingredient:	Pregnancy Risk Category:
Bisacodyl	C

Helpful Hints and Reminders: Each pregnancy risk category (**A**, **B**, **C**, **D**, or **X**) is explained on the last page of this section.

Remember: All pregnancies have a background risk of 3% or more for a serious birth defect, even when mom doesn't take a drug of any kind. If you are pregnant or planning a pregnancy, always let your healthcare provider know before taking any drug, prescription or non-prescription, or herbal remedy.

Dulcolax® Stool Softener

Active Ingredient:	Pregnancy Risk Category:
Docusate sodium	C

Helpful Hints and Reminders: Each pregnancy risk category (**A**, **B**, **C**, **D**, or **X**) is explained on the last page of this section.

Remember: All pregnancies have a background risk of 3% or more for a serious birth defect, even when mom doesn't take a drug of any kind. If you are pregnant or planning a pregnancy, always let your healthcare provider know before taking any drug, prescription or non-prescription, or herbal remedy.

Equate® Clear Lax Polyethylene Glycol 3350 Laxative

Active Ingredient:	Pregnancy Risk Category:
Polyethylene glycol 3350	C

Helpful Hints and Reminders: Each pregnancy risk category (**A**, **B**, **C**, **D**, or **X**) is explained on the last page of this section.

Remember: All pregnancies have a background risk of 3% or more for a serious birth defect, even when mom doesn't take a drug of any kind. If you are pregnant or planning a pregnancy, always let your healthcare provider know before taking any drug, prescription or non-prescription, or herbal remedy.

Equate® Docusate Sodium Stool Softener Softgels

Active Ingredient:	Pregnancy Risk Category:
Docusate sodium	C

Helpful Hints and Reminders: Each pregnancy risk category (**A**, **B**, **C**, **D**, or **X**) is explained on the last page of this section.

Remember: All pregnancies have a background risk of 3% or more for a serious birth defect, even when mom doesn't take a drug of any kind. If you are pregnant or planning a pregnancy, always let your healthcare provider know before taking any drug, prescription or non-prescription, or herbal remedy.

Equate® Laxative Fiber Therapy Caplets

Active Ingredient:	Pregnancy Risk Category:
Methylcellulose	C

Helpful Hints and Reminders: Each pregnancy risk category (**A**, **B**, **C**, **D**, or **X**) is explained on the last page of this section.

Remember: All pregnancies have a background risk of 3% or more for a serious birth defect, even when mom doesn't take a drug of any kind. If you are pregnant or planning a pregnancy, always let your healthcare provider know before taking any drug, prescription or non-prescription, or herbal remedy.

Equate® Maximum Strength Laxative Pills

Active Ingredient:	Pregnancy Risk Category:
Sennosides	C

Helpful Hints and Reminders: Each pregnancy risk category (**A**, **B**, **C**, **D**, or **X**) is explained on the last page of this section.

Remember: All pregnancies have a background risk of 3% or more for a serious birth defect, even when mom doesn't take a drug of any kind. If you are pregnant or planning a pregnancy, always let your healthcare provider know before taking any drug, prescription or non-prescription, or herbal remedy.

Equate® Stimulant Laxative 5 Mg Tablets

Active Ingredient:	Pregnancy Risk Category:
Bisacodyl	C

Helpful Hints and Reminders: Each pregnancy risk category (**A**, **B**, **C**, **D**, or **X**) is explained on the last page of this section.

Remember: All pregnancies have a background risk of 3% or more for a serious birth defect, even when mom doesn't take a drug of any kind. If you are pregnant or planning a pregnancy, always let your healthcare provider know before taking any drug, prescription or non-prescription, or herbal remedy.

Equate® Women's Bisacodyl Stimulant Laxative Tablets

Active Ingredient:	Pregnancy Risk Category:
Bisacodyl	C

Helpful Hints and Reminders: Each pregnancy risk category (**A**, **B**, **C**, **D**, or **X**) is explained on the last page of this section.

Remember: All pregnancies have a background risk of 3% or more for a serious birth defect, even when mom doesn't take a drug of any kind.

If you are pregnant or planning a pregnancy, always let your healthcare provider know before taking any drug, prescription or non-prescription, or herbal remedy.

Ex-Lax® Chocolated Stimulant Laxative

Active Ingredient:	Pregnancy Risk Category:
Sennosides	C

Helpful Hints and Reminders: Each pregnancy risk category (**A**, **B**, **C**, **D**, or **X**) is explained on the last page of this section.

Remember: All pregnancies have a background risk of 3% or more for a serious birth defect, even when mom doesn't take a drug of any kind. If you are pregnant or planning a pregnancy, always let your healthcare provider know before taking any drug, prescription or non-prescription, or herbal remedy.

Ex-Lax® Laxative Pills, Regular & Maximum Strength

Active Ingredient:	Pregnancy Risk Category:
Sennosides	C

Helpful Hints and Reminders: Each pregnancy risk category (**A**, **B**, **C**, **D**, or **X**) is explained on the last page of this section.

Remember: All pregnancies have a background risk of 3% or more for a serious birth defect, even when mom doesn't take a drug of any kind. If you are pregnant or planning a pregnancy, always let your healthcare provider know before taking any drug, prescription or non-prescription, or herbal remedy.

Fibercon Caplets: Bulk-Forming Laxative

Active Ingredient:	Pregnancy Risk Category:
Calcium polycarbophil	C

Helpful Hints and Reminders: Each pregnancy risk category (**A**, **B**, **C**, **D**, or **X**) is explained on the last page of this section.

Remember: All pregnancies have a background risk of 3% or more for a serious birth defect, even when mom doesn't take a drug of any kind. If you are pregnant or planning a pregnancy, always let your healthcare provider know before taking any drug, prescription or non-prescription, or herbal remedy.

Kirkland Signature™ Fiber Tabs Bulk-Forming Fiber Laxative

Active Ingredient:	Pregnancy Risk Category:
Calcium polycarbophil	C

Helpful Hints and Reminders: Each pregnancy risk category (**A**, **B**, **C**, **D**, or **X**) is explained on the last page of this section.

Remember: All pregnancies have a background risk of 3% or more for a serious birth defect, even when mom doesn't take a drug of any kind. If you are pregnant or planning a pregnancy, always let your healthcare provider know before taking any drug, prescription or non-prescription, or herbal remedy.

Metamucil® Fiber Laxative: Powders, Capsules & Wafers

Active Ingredient:	Pregnancy Risk Category:
Psyllium husk	B

Helpful Hints and Reminders: Each pregnancy risk category (**A**, **B**, **C**, **D**, or **X**) is explained on the last page of this section.

Remember: All pregnancies have a background risk of 3% or more for a serious birth defect, even when mom doesn't take a drug of any kind. If you are pregnant or planning a pregnancy, always let your healthcare provider know before taking any drug, prescription or non-prescription, or herbal remedy.

MiraLAX® Powder Laxative

Active Ingredient:	Pregnancy Risk Category:
Polyethylene glycol 3350	C

Helpful Hints and Reminders: Each pregnancy risk category (**A**, **B**, **C**, **D**, or **X**) is explained on the last page of this section.

Remember: All pregnancies have a background risk of 3% or more for a serious birth defect, even when mom doesn't take a drug of any kind. If you are pregnant or planning a pregnancy, always let your healthcare provider know before taking any drug, prescription or non-prescription, or herbal remedy.

Peri-Colace® Tablets

Active Ingredients:	Pregnancy Risk Category:
Docusate sodium	C
Sennosides	C

Helpful Hints and Reminders: Each pregnancy risk category (**A**, **B**, **C**, **D**, or **X**) is explained on the last page of this section.

Remember: All pregnancies have a background risk of 3% or more for a serious birth defect, even when mom doesn't take a drug of any kind. If you are pregnant or planning a pregnancy, always let your healthcare provider know before taking any drug, prescription or non-prescription, or herbal remedy.

Phillips® Genuine Laxative Caplets

Active Ingredient:	Pregnancy Risk Category:
Magnesium oxide	**Risk is undetermined**. The FDA has not assigned a pregnancy risk category to this drug. However, magnesium oxide is approved by the FDA as a magnesium supplement during pregnancy.

Helpful Hints and Reminders: Each pregnancy risk category (**A**, **B**, **C**, **D**, or **X**) is explained on the last page of this section.

Remember: All pregnancies have a background risk of 3% or more for a serious birth defect, even when mom doesn't take a drug of any kind. If you are pregnant or planning a pregnancy, always let your healthcare provider know before taking any drug, prescription or non-prescription, or herbal remedy.

Phillips® Genuine Milk of Magnesia

Active Ingredient:	Pregnancy Risk Category:
Magnesium hydroxide	C

Helpful Hints and Reminders: Each pregnancy risk category (**A**, **B**, **C**, **D**, or **X**) is explained on the last page of this section.

Remember: All pregnancies have a background risk of 3% or more for a serious birth defect, even when mom doesn't take a drug of any kind. If you are pregnant or planning a pregnancy, always let your healthcare provider know before taking any drug, prescription or non-prescription, or herbal remedy.

Target® Maximum Strength Laxative Tablets

Active Ingredient:	Pregnancy Risk Category:
Sennosides	C

Helpful Hints and Reminders: Each pregnancy risk category (**A**, **B**, **C**, **D**, or **X**) is explained on the last page of this section.

Remember: All pregnancies have a background risk of 3% or more for a serious birth defect, even when mom doesn't take a drug of any kind. If you are pregnant or planning a pregnancy, always let your healthcare provider know before taking any drug, prescription or non-prescription, or herbal remedy.

Target® Stool Softener & Stimulant Laxative Tablets

Active Ingredients:	Pregnancy Risk Category:
Docusate sodium	C
Sennosides	C

Helpful Hints and Reminders: Each pregnancy risk category (**A**, **B**, **C**, **D**, or **X**) is explained on the last page of this section.

Remember: All pregnancies have a background risk of 3% or more for a serious birth defect, even when mom doesn't take a drug of any kind. If you are pregnant or planning a pregnancy, always let your healthcare provider know before taking any drug, prescription or non-prescription, or herbal remedy.

Target® Stool Softener Soft Gels

Active Ingredient:	Pregnancy Risk Category:
Docusate sodium	C

Helpful Hints and Reminders: Each pregnancy risk category (**A**, **B**, **C**, **D**, or **X**) is explained on the last page of this section.

Remember: All pregnancies have a background risk of 3% or more for a serious birth defect, even when mom doesn't take a drug of any kind. If you are pregnant or planning a pregnancy, always let your healthcare provider know before taking any drug, prescription or non-prescription, or herbal remedy.

Target® Sugar-Free Fiber Therapy Laxative Powder

Active Ingredient:	Pregnancy Risk Category:
Psyllium husk	B

Helpful Hints and Reminders: Each pregnancy risk category (**A**, **B**, **C**, **D**, or **X**) is explained on the last page of this section.

Target® Women's Laxative Tablets

Remember: All pregnancies have a background risk of 3% or more for a serious birth defect, even when mom doesn't take a drug of any kind. If you are pregnant or planning a pregnancy, always let your healthcare provider know before taking any drug, prescription or non-prescription, or herbal remedy.

Target® Women's Laxative Tablets

Active Ingredient:	Pregnancy Risk Category:
Bisacodyl	C

Helpful Hints and Reminders: Each pregnancy risk category (**A**, **B**, **C**, **D**, or **X**) is explained on the last page of this section.

Remember: All pregnancies have a background risk of 3% or more for a serious birth defect, even when mom doesn't take a drug of any kind. If you are pregnant or planning a pregnancy, always let your healthcare provider know before taking any drug, prescription or non-prescription, or herbal remedy.

The FDA's Pregnancy Risk Categories: A, B, C, D, X

Adapted to the Active Ingredients in Nonprescription drugs

Category A: Controlled studies using the active ingredient in pregnant women have not shown harmful fetal effects throughout pregnancy, and the possibility of fetal harm seems remote. My comment: *Though apparently safe, these active ingredients should still only be used in pregnancy when clearly indicated.*

Category B: Either studies have shown no evidence of fetal harm when using the active ingredient in pregnant animals, but no controlled studies have been done in pregnant women, **or** studies have shown evidence of fetal harm when using the active ingredient in pregnant animals, but controlled studies in pregnant women have not shown evidence of fetal harm. My comment: *These active ingredients should only be used in pregnancy when clearly indicated.*

Category C: Either studies have shown evidence of fetal harm when using the active ingredient in pregnant animals, but no controlled studies have been done in pregnant women, **or** studies using the active ingredient in pregnant animals have not been done, and studies of pregnant women are insufficient to reach a conclusion. These active ingredients should only be used by a pregnant woman if the potential benefit justifies the potential risk of fetal harm, which, in many cases, is unknown. My comment: *It's impossible to calculate the potential risk of fetal harm when, in many cases, it's unknown. Thus, these active ingredients should only be used in pregnancy when clearly needed.*

Category D: Studies have shown evidence of fetal harm when using the active ingredient in pregnant women. However, the potential benefit of using the active ingredient in some life-threatening situations for

mom may outweigh the potential risk of fetal harm. For example, when mom requires cancer treatment or when she has a serious disease for which safer active ingredients cannot be used or are less effective. My comment: *These exceptional indications rarely occur when considering a nonprescription drug in pregnancy.*

Category X: My comment: *Because the risk of fetal harm is too high, no Category X active ingredients have been approved for use in nonprescription drugs.*

Active Ingredients Assigned Two Pregnancy Risk Categories: Some active ingredients have two pregnancy risk categories, depending on which trimester of pregnancy the active ingredient is used. For example, naproxen sodium, the active ingredient in Aleve, belongs to Category **B** when used in the first and second trimesters of pregnancy. If used in the third trimester, however, the active ingredient belongs to Category **D**. My comment: *This means naproxen sodium should not be used in the third trimester unless prescribed by a physician who has advised her patient of the risks involved.*

Section 4: Diarrhea

CVS® Anti-Diarrheal Caplets

Active Ingredient:	Pregnancy Risk Category:
Loperamide Hcl	B

Helpful Hints and Reminders: Each pregnancy risk category (**A**, **B**, **C**, **D**, or **X**) is explained on the last page of this section.

Remember: All pregnancies have a background risk of 3% or more for a serious birth defect, even when mom doesn't take a drug of any kind. If you are pregnant or planning a pregnancy, always let your healthcare provider know before taking any drug, prescription or non-prescription, or herbal remedy.

CVS® Stomach Relief Caplets

Active Ingredient:	Pregnancy Risk Category:
Bismuth subsalicylate	C (See Helpful Hints below.)

Helpful Hints and Reminders: Each pregnancy risk category (**A**, **B**, **C**, **D**, or **X**) is explained on the last page of this section.

1. "Although the risk of harm may be small, significant adverse fetal effects have resulted from chronic exposure to salicylates. Because of this, the use of bismuth subsalicylate during pregnancy

Equate® Antacid Pink-Bismuth Tablets

should be restricted to the first half, and then only in amounts that do not exceed the recommended doses," according to G. G. Briggs et al, "Drugs in Pregnancy and Lactation." (See Reference Section in the Appendix.)

Remember: All pregnancies have a background risk of 3% or more for a serious birth defect, even when mom doesn't take a drug of any kind. If you are pregnant or planning a pregnancy, always let your healthcare provider know before taking any drug, prescription or non-prescription, or herbal remedy.

CVS® Stomach Relief Liquid Maximum Strength

Active Ingredient:	Pregnancy Risk Category:
Bismuth subsalicylate	C (See Helpful Hints below.)

Helpful Hints and Reminders: Each pregnancy risk category (**A**, **B**, **C**, **D**, or **X**) is explained on the last page of this section.

1. "Although the risk of harm may be small, significant adverse fetal effects have resulted from chronic exposure to salicylates. Because of this, the use of bismuth subsalicylate during pregnancy should be restricted to the first half, and then only in amounts that do not exceed the recommended doses," according to G. G. Briggs et al, "Drugs in Pregnancy and Lactation." (See Reference Section in the Appendix.)

Remember: All pregnancies have a background risk of 3% or more for a serious birth defect, even when mom doesn't take a drug of any kind. If you are pregnant or planning a pregnancy, always let your healthcare provider know before taking any drug, prescription or non-prescription, or herbal remedy.

Equate® Antacid Pink-Bismuth Tablets

Active Ingredient:	Pregnancy Risk Category:
Bismuth subsalicylate	C (See Helpful Hints on the next page.)

Helpful Hints and Reminders: Each pregnancy risk category (**A**, **B**, **C**, **D**, or **X**) is explained on the last page of this section.

1. "Although the risk of harm may be small, significant adverse fetal effects have resulted from chronic exposure to salicylates. Because of this, the use of bismuth subsalicylate during pregnancy should be restricted to the first half, and then only in amounts that do not exceed the recommended doses," according to G. G. Briggs et al, "Drugs in Pregnancy and Lactation." (See Reference Section in the Appendix.)

Remember: All pregnancies have a background risk of 3% or more for a serious birth defect, even when mom doesn't take a drug of any kind. If you are pregnant or planning a pregnancy, always let your healthcare provider know before taking any drug, prescription or non-prescription, or herbal remedy.

Equate® Anti-Diarrheal Caplets

Active Ingredient:	Pregnancy Risk Category:
Loperamide Hcl	B

Helpful Hints and Reminders: Each pregnancy risk category (**A**, **B**, **C**, **D**, or **X**) is explained on the last page of this section.

Remember: All pregnancies have a background risk of 3% or more for a serious birth defect, even when mom doesn't take a drug of any kind. If you are pregnant or planning a pregnancy, always let your healthcare provider know before taking any drug, prescription or non-prescription, or herbal remedy.

Equate® Loperamide Hydrochloride Tablets 2 Mg Anti-Diarrheal

Active Ingredient:	Pregnancy Risk Category:
Loperamide Hcl	B

Helpful Hints and Reminders: Each pregnancy risk category (**A**, **B**, **C**, **D**, or **X**) is explained on the last page of this section.

Remember: All pregnancies have a background risk of 3% or more for a serious birth defect, even when mom doesn't take a drug of any kind. If you are pregnant or planning a pregnancy, always let your healthcare provider know before taking any drug, prescription or non-prescription, or herbal remedy.

Imodium® A-D, Caplets & Mint-Flavored Liquid

Active Ingredient:	Pregnancy Risk Category:
Loperamide Hcl	B

Helpful Hints and Reminders: Each pregnancy risk category (**A**, **B**, **C**, **D**, or **X**) is explained on the last page of this section.

Remember: All pregnancies have a background risk of 3% or more for a serious birth defect, even when mom doesn't take a drug of any kind. If you are pregnant or planning a pregnancy, always let your healthcare provider know before taking any drug, prescription or non-prescription, or herbal remedy.

Imodium® A-D, EZ Chews

Active Ingredient:	Pregnancy Risk Category:
Loperamide Hcl	B

Helpful Hints and Reminders: Each pregnancy risk category (**A**, **B**, **C**, **D**, or **X**) is explained on the last page of this section.

Remember: All pregnancies have a background risk of 3% or more for a serious birth defect, even when mom doesn't take a drug of any kind. If you are pregnant or planning a pregnancy, always let your healthcare provider know before taking any drug, prescription or non-prescription, or herbal remedy.

Imodium® Multi-Symptom Relief, Chewable Tablets & Caplets

Active Ingredient:	Pregnancy Risk Category:
Loperamide Hcl	B
Simethicone	C

Helpful Hints and Reminders: Each pregnancy risk category (**A**, **B**, **C**, **D**, or **X**) is explained on the last page of this section.

Remember: All pregnancies have a background risk of 3% or more for a serious birth defect, even when mom doesn't take a drug of any kind. If you are pregnant or planning a pregnancy, always let your healthcare provider know before taking any drug, prescription or non-prescription, or herbal remedy.

Kirkland Signature™ Anti-Diarrheal

Active Ingredient:	Pregnancy Risk Category:
Loperamide Hcl	B

Helpful Hints and Reminders: Each pregnancy risk category (**A**, **B**, **C**, **D**, or **X**) is explained on the last page of this section.

Remember: All pregnancies have a background risk of 3% or more for a serious birth defect, even when mom doesn't take a drug of any kind. If you are pregnant or planning a pregnancy, always let your healthcare provider know before taking any drug, prescription or non-prescription, or herbal remedy.

Up & Up™ Bismuth Stomach Relief

Active Ingredient:	Pregnancy Risk Category:
Bismuth subsalicylate	C (See Helpful Hints below.)

Helpful Hints and Reminders: Each pregnancy risk category (**A**, **B**, **C**, **D**, or **X**) is explained on the last page of this section.

1. "Although the risk of harm may be small, significant adverse fetal effects have resulted from chronic exposure to salicylates. Because of this, the use of bismuth subsalicylate during pregnancy should be restricted to the first half, and then only in amounts that do not exceed the recommended doses," according to G. G. Briggs et al, "Drugs in Pregnancy and Lactation." (See Reference Section in the Appendix.)

Remember: All pregnancies have a background risk of 3% or more for a serious birth defect, even when mom doesn't take a drug of any kind. If you are pregnant or planning a pregnancy, always let your healthcare provider know before taking any drug, prescription or non-prescription, or herbal remedy.

The FDA's Pregnancy Risk Categories: A, B, C, D, X

Adapted to the Active Ingredients in Nonprescription drugs

Category A: Controlled studies using the active ingredient in pregnant women have not shown harmful fetal effects throughout pregnancy, and the possibility of fetal harm seems remote. My comment: *Though apparently safe, these active ingredients should still only be used in pregnancy when clearly indicated.*

Category B: Either studies have shown no evidence of fetal harm when using the active ingredient in pregnant animals, but no controlled studies have been done in pregnant women, **or** studies have shown evidence of fetal harm when using the active ingredient in pregnant animals, but controlled studies in pregnant women have not shown evidence of fetal harm. My comment: *These active ingredients should only be used in pregnancy when clearly indicated.*

Category C: Either studies have shown evidence of fetal harm when using the active ingredient in pregnant animals, but no controlled studies have been done in pregnant women, **or** studies using the active ingredient in pregnant animals have not been done, and studies of pregnant women are insufficient to reach a conclusion. These active ingredients should only be used by a pregnant woman if the potential benefit justifies the potential risk of fetal harm, which, in many cases, is unknown. My comment: *It's impossible to calculate the potential risk of fetal harm when, in many cases, it's unknown. Thus, these active ingredients should only be used in pregnancy when clearly needed.*

Category D: Studies have shown evidence of fetal harm when using the active ingredient in pregnant women. However, the potential benefit of using the active ingredient in some life-threatening situations for

mom may outweigh the potential risk of fetal harm. For example, when mom requires cancer treatment or when she has a serious disease for which safer active ingredients cannot be used or are less effective. My comment: *These exceptional indications rarely occur when considering a nonprescription drug in pregnancy.*

Category X: My comment: *Because the risk of fetal harm is too high, no Category X active ingredients have been approved for use in nonprescription drugs.*

Active Ingredients Assigned Two Pregnancy Risk Categories: Some active ingredients have two pregnancy risk categories, depending on which trimester of pregnancy the active ingredient is used. For example, naproxen sodium, the active ingredient in Aleve, belongs to Category **B** when used in the first and second trimesters of pregnancy. If used in the third trimester, however, the active ingredient belongs to Category **D**. My comment: *This means naproxen sodium should not be used in the third trimester unless prescribed by a physician who has advised her patient of the risks involved.*

Section 5: Fungal, Yeast, & Other Infections

Abreva® Pump & Original Tube

Active Ingredient:	Pregnancy Risk Category:
Docosanol	B

Helpful Hints and Reminders: Each pregnancy risk category (**A**, **B**, **C**, **D**, or **X**) is explained on the last page of this section.

Remember: All pregnancies have a background risk of 3% or more for a serious birth defect, even when mom doesn't take a drug of any kind. If you are pregnant or planning a pregnancy, always let your healthcare provider know before taking any drug, prescription or non-prescription, or herbal remedy.

....

Desenex® Antifungal (Shake Powder, Liquid Spray, Spray Powder, Jock Itch Spray & Powder)

Active Ingredient:	Pregnancy Risk Category:
Miconazole 2%	C

Helpful Hints and Reminders: Each pregnancy risk category (**A**, **B**, **C**, **D**, or **X**) is explained on the last page of this section.

Remember: All pregnancies have a background risk of 3% or more for a serious birth defect, even when mom doesn't take a drug of any kind. If you are pregnant or planning a pregnancy, always let your healthcare provider know before taking any drug, prescription or non-prescription, or herbal remedy.

Desenex® Cream

Active Ingredient:	Pregnancy Risk Category:
Clotrimazole 1%	B

Helpful Hints and Reminders: Each pregnancy risk category (**A**, **B**, **C**, **D**, or **X**) is explained on the last page of this section.

Remember: All pregnancies have a background risk of 3% or more for a serious birth defect, even when mom doesn't take a drug of any kind. If you are pregnant or planning a pregnancy, always let your healthcare provider know before taking any drug, prescription or non-prescription, or herbal remedy.

Equate® Povidone-Iodine Solution, 10% Topical Microbicide Antiseptic

Active Ingredient:	Pregnancy Risk Category:
Povidone-Iodine, 10%	D

Helpful Hints and Reminders: Each pregnancy risk category (**A**, **B**, **C**, **D**, or **X**) is explained on the last page of this section.

Remember: All pregnancies have a background risk of 3% or more for a serious birth defect, even when mom doesn't take a drug of any kind. If you are pregnant or planning a pregnancy, always let your healthcare provider know before taking any drug, prescription or non-prescription, or herbal remedy.

Lamisil AF Defense®: Shake Powder & Spray Powder

Active Ingredient:	Pregnancy Risk Category:
Tolnaftate	C

Helpful Hints and Reminders: Each pregnancy risk category (**A**, **B**, **C**, **D**, or **X**) is explained on the last page of this section.

Remember: All pregnancies have a background risk of 3% or more for a serious birth defect, even when mom doesn't take a drug of any kind. If you are pregnant or planning a pregnancy, always let your healthcare provider know before taking any drug, prescription or non-prescription, or herbal remedy.

Lamisil AT® Cream

Active Ingredient:	Pregnancy Risk Category:
Terbinafine Hcl	B

Helpful Hints and Reminders: Each pregnancy risk category (**A**, **B**, **C**, **D**, or **X**) is explained on the last page of this section.

Remember: All pregnancies have a background risk of 3% or more for a serious birth defect, even when mom doesn't take a drug of any kind. If you are pregnant or planning a pregnancy, always let your healthcare provider know before taking any drug, prescription or non-prescription, or herbal remedy.

Neosporin® First Aid Antibiotic Ointment

Active Ingredient:	Pregnancy Risk Category:
Polymyxin B sulfate	B
Bacitracin zinc	C
Neomycin	C

Helpful Hints and Reminders: Each pregnancy risk category (**A**, **B**, **C**, **D**, or **X**) is explained on the last page of this section.

Remember: All pregnancies have a background risk of 3% or more for a serious birth defect, even when mom doesn't take a drug of any kind. If you are pregnant or planning a pregnancy, always let your healthcare provider know before taking any drug, prescription or non-prescription, or herbal remedy.

Neosporin® First Aid Antiseptic/ Pain Relieving Spray

Active Ingredient:	Pregnancy Risk Category:
Pramoxine Hcl	C
Benzalkonium chloride	**Risk is undetermined.** The FDA has not assigned a pregnancy risk category to this drug.

Helpful Hints and Reminders: Each pregnancy risk category (**A**, **B**, **C**, **D**, or **X**) is explained on the last page of this section.

Remember: All pregnancies have a background risk of 3% or more for a serious birth defect, even when mom doesn't take a drug of any kind. If you are pregnant or planning a pregnancy, always let your healthcare provider know before taking any drug, prescription or non-prescription, or herbal remedy.

Neosporin® Plus Pain Relief, Maximum Strength, First Aid Antibiotic Cream

Active Ingredient:	Pregnancy Risk Category:
Polymyxin B sulfate	B
Neomycin	C
Pramoxine Hcl	C

Helpful Hints and Reminders: Each pregnancy risk category (**A**, **B**, **C**, **D**, or **X**) is explained on the last page of this section.

Remember: All pregnancies have a background risk of 3% or more for a serious birth defect, even when mom doesn't take a drug of any kind. If you are pregnant or planning a pregnancy, always let your healthcare

provider know before taking any drug, prescription or non-prescription, or herbal remedy.

Permethrin Lotion 1%

Active Ingredient:	Pregnancy Risk Category:
Permethrin	B

Helpful Hints and Reminders: Each pregnancy risk category (**A**, **B**, **C**, **D**, or **X**) is explained on the last page of this section.

Remember: All pregnancies have a background risk of 3% or more for a serious birth defect, even when mom doesn't take a drug of any kind. If you are pregnant or planning a pregnancy, always let your healthcare provider know before taking any drug, prescription or non-prescription, or herbal remedy.

Polysporin® First Aid Antibiotic Ointment

Active Ingredient:	Pregnancy Risk Category:
Bacitracin	C
Polymyxin B	B

Helpful Hints and Reminders: Each pregnancy risk category (**A**, **B**, **C**, **D**, or **X**) is explained on the last page of this section.

Remember: All pregnancies have a background risk of 3% or more for a serious birth defect, even when mom doesn't take a drug of any kind. If you are pregnant or planning a pregnancy, always let your healthcare provider know before taking any drug, prescription or non-prescription, or herbal remedy.

Polysporin® First Aid Antibiotic Powder

Active Ingredient:	Pregnancy Risk Category:
Bacitracin	C
Polymyxin B	B

Helpful Hints and Reminders: Each pregnancy risk category (**A**, **B**, **C**, **D**, or **X**) is explained on the last page of this section.

Remember: All pregnancies have a background risk of 3% or more for a serious birth defect, even when mom doesn't take a drug of any kind. If you are pregnant or planning a pregnancy, always let your healthcare provider know before taking any drug, prescription or non-prescription, or herbal remedy.

Rite Aid® Athlete's Foot Cream Clotrimazole 1% Cream

Active Ingredient:	Pregnancy Risk Category:
Clotrimazole	B

Helpful Hints and Reminders: Each pregnancy risk category (**A**, **B**, **C**, **D**, or **X**) is explained on the last page of this section.

Remember: All pregnancies have a background risk of 3% or more for a serious birth defect, even when mom doesn't take a drug of any kind. If you are pregnant or planning a pregnancy, always let your healthcare provider know before taking any drug, prescription or non-prescription, or herbal remedy.

Target® Antifungal Foot Spray

Active Ingredient:	Pregnancy Risk Category:
Tolnaftate	C

Helpful Hints and Reminders: Each pregnancy risk category (**A**, **B**, **C**, **D**, or **X**) is explained on the last page of this section.

Remember: All pregnancies have a background risk of 3% or more for a serious birth defect, even when mom doesn't take a drug of any kind. If you are pregnant or planning a pregnancy, always let your healthcare provider know before taking any drug, prescription or non-prescription, or herbal remedy.

Target® Athlete's Foot Cream

Active Ingredient:	Pregnancy Risk Category:
Terbinafine Hcl	B

Helpful Hints and Reminders: Each pregnancy risk category (**A**, **B**, **C**, **D**, or **X**) is explained on the last page of this section.

Remember: All pregnancies have a background risk of 3% or more for a serious birth defect, even when mom doesn't take a drug of any kind. If you are pregnant or planning a pregnancy, always let your healthcare provider know before taking any drug, prescription or non-prescription, or herbal remedy.

Vagistat-1 (Tioconazole Ointment 6.5%)

Active Ingredient:	Pregnancy Risk Category:
Tioconazole	C

Helpful Hints and Reminders: Each pregnancy risk category (**A**, **B**, **C**, **D**, or **X**) is explained on the last page of this section.

Remember: All pregnancies have a background risk of 3% or more for a serious birth defect, even when mom doesn't take a drug of any kind. If you are pregnant or planning a pregnancy, always let your healthcare provider know before taking any drug, prescription or non-prescription, or herbal remedy.

The FDA's Pregnancy Risk Categories: A, B, C, D, X

Adapted to the Active Ingredients in Nonprescription drugs

Category A: Controlled studies using the active ingredient in pregnant women have not shown harmful fetal effects throughout pregnancy, and the possibility of fetal harm seems remote. My comment: *Though apparently safe, these active ingredients should still only be used in pregnancy when clearly indicated.*

Category B: Either studies have shown no evidence of fetal harm when using the active ingredient in pregnant animals, but no controlled studies have been done in pregnant women, **or** studies have shown evidence of fetal harm when using the active ingredient in pregnant animals, but controlled studies in pregnant women have not shown evidence of fetal harm. My comment: *These active ingredients should only be used in pregnancy when clearly indicated.*

Category C: Either studies have shown evidence of fetal harm when using the active ingredient in pregnant animals, but no controlled studies have been done in pregnant women, **or** studies using the active ingredient in pregnant animals have not been done, and studies of pregnant women are insufficient to reach a conclusion. These active ingredients should only be used by a pregnant woman if the potential benefit justifies the potential risk of fetal harm, which, in many cases, is unknown. My comment: *It's impossible to calculate the potential risk of fetal harm when, in many cases, it's unknown. Thus, these active ingredients should only be used in pregnancy when clearly needed.*

Category D: Studies have shown evidence of fetal harm when using the active ingredient in pregnant women. However, the potential benefit of using the active ingredient in some life-threatening situations for

mom may outweigh the potential risk of fetal harm. For example, when mom requires cancer treatment or when she has a serious disease for which safer active ingredients cannot be used or are less effective. My comment: *These exceptional indications rarely occur when considering a nonprescription drug in pregnancy.*

Category X: My comment: *Because the risk of fetal harm is too high, no Category X active ingredients have been approved for use in nonprescription drugs.*

Active Ingredients Assigned Two Pregnancy Risk Categories: Some active ingredients have two pregnancy risk categories, depending on which trimester of pregnancy the active ingredient is used. For example, naproxen sodium, the active ingredient in Aleve, belongs to Category **B** when used in the first and second trimesters of pregnancy. If used in the third trimester, however, the active ingredient belongs to Category **D**. My comment: *This means naproxen sodium should not be used in the third trimester unless prescribed by a physician who has advised her patient of the risks involved.*

Section 6: Gas

Equate® Extra Strength Gas Relief Chewable Tablets

Active Ingredient:	Pregnancy Risk Category:
Simethicone	C

Helpful Hints and Reminders: Each pregnancy risk category (**A**, **B**, **C**, **D**, or **X**) is explained on the last page of this section.

Remember: All pregnancies have a background risk of 3% or more for a serious birth defect, even when mom doesn't take a drug of any kind. If you are pregnant or planning a pregnancy, always let your healthcare provider know before taking any drug, prescription or non-prescription, or herbal remedy.

Equate® Liquid Maximum Strength Original Classic Antacid/Anti-Gas

Active Ingredient:	Pregnancy Risk Category:
Aluminum hydroxide	C
Magnesium hydroxide	C
Simethicone	C

Helpful Hints and Reminders: Each pregnancy risk category (**A**, **B**, **C**, **D**, or **X**) is explained on the last page of this section.

Remember: All pregnancies have a background risk of 3% or more for a serious birth defect, even when mom doesn't take a drug of any kind. If you are pregnant or planning a pregnancy, always let your healthcare provider know before taking any drug, prescription or non-prescription, or herbal remedy.

Equate® Regular Strength Liquid Cooling Mint Antacid/Anti-Gas

Active Ingredient:	Pregnancy Risk Category:
Aluminum hydroxide	C
Magnesium hydroxide	C
Simethicone	C

Helpful Hints and Reminders: Each pregnancy risk category (**A**, **B**, **C**, **D**, or **X**) is explained on the last page of this section.

Remember: All pregnancies have a background risk of 3% or more for a serious birth defect, even when mom doesn't take a drug of any kind. If you are pregnant or planning a pregnancy, always let your healthcare provider know before taking any drug, prescription or non-prescription, or herbal remedy.

Gas-X® Extra Strength: Antigas Softgels & Chewable Tablets

Active Ingredient:	Pregnancy Risk Category:
Simethicone	C

Helpful Hints and Reminders: Each pregnancy risk category (**A**, **B**, **C**, **D**, or **X**) is explained on the last page of this section.

Remember: All pregnancies have a background risk of 3% or more for a serious birth defect, even when mom doesn't take a drug of any kind. If you are pregnant or planning a pregnancy, always let your healthcare

provider know before taking any drug, prescription or non-prescription, or herbal remedy.

Gas-X® Maximum Strength: Antigas Softgels

Active Ingredient:	Pregnancy Risk Category:
Simethicone	C

Helpful Hints and Reminders: Each pregnancy risk category (**A**, **B**, **C**, **D**, or **X**) is explained on the last page of this section.

Remember: All pregnancies have a background risk of 3% or more for a serious birth defect, even when mom doesn't take a drug of any kind. If you are pregnant or planning a pregnancy, always let your healthcare provider know before taking any drug, prescription or non-prescription, or herbal remedy.

Gas-X® Regular Strength: Antigas Chewable Tablets

Active Ingredient:	Pregnancy Risk Category:
Simethicone	C

Helpful Hints and Reminders: Each pregnancy risk category (**A**, **B**, **C**, **D**, or **X**) is explained on the last page of this section.

Remember: All pregnancies have a background risk of 3% or more for a serious birth defect, even when mom doesn't take a drug of any kind. If you are pregnant or planning a pregnancy, always let your healthcare provider know before taking any drug, prescription or non-prescription, or herbal remedy.

Gas-X® Thin Strips

Active Ingredient:	Pregnancy Risk Category:
Simethicone	C

Helpful Hints and Reminders: Each pregnancy risk category (**A**, **B**, **C**, **D**, or **X**) is explained on the last page of this section.

Remember: All pregnancies have a background risk of 3% or more for a serious birth defect, even when mom doesn't take a drug of any kind. If you are pregnant or planning a pregnancy, always let your healthcare provider know before taking any drug, prescription or non-prescription, or herbal remedy.

Gas-X® with Maalox Extra Strength: Chewable Tablets

Active Ingredient:	Pregnancy Risk Category:
Simethicone	C
Calcium carbonate	C

Helpful Hints and Reminders: Each pregnancy risk category (**A**, **B**, **C**, **D**, or **X**) is explained on the last page of this section.

Remember: All pregnancies have a background risk of 3% or more for a serious birth defect, even when mom doesn't take a drug of any kind. If you are pregnant or planning a pregnancy, always let your healthcare provider know before taking any drug, prescription or non-prescription, or herbal remedy.

Gelusil® Antacid/Anti-Gas Tablets

Active Ingredient:	Pregnancy Risk Category:
Aluminum hydroxide	C
Magnesium hydroxide	C
Simethicone	C

Helpful Hints and Reminders: Each pregnancy risk category (**A**, **B**, **C**, **D**, or **X**) is explained on the last page of this section.

Remember: All pregnancies have a background risk of 3% or more for a serious birth defect, even when mom doesn't take a drug of any kind. If you are pregnant or planning a pregnancy, always let your healthcare

provider know before taking any drug, prescription or non-prescription, or herbal remedy.

Mylanta® Gas Maximum Strength Chewable Tablets

Active Ingredient:	Pregnancy Risk Category:
Simethicone	C

Helpful Hints and Reminders: Each pregnancy risk category (**A**, **B**, **C**, **D**, or **X**) is explained on the last page of this section.

Remember: All pregnancies have a background risk of 3% or more for a serious birth defect, even when mom doesn't take a drug of any kind. If you are pregnant or planning a pregnancy, always let your healthcare provider know before taking any drug, prescription or non-prescription, or herbal remedy.

Mylanta® Gas Maximum Strength Softgels

Active Ingredient:	Pregnancy Risk Category:
Simethicone	C

Helpful Hints and Reminders: Each pregnancy risk category (**A**, **B**, **C**, **D**, or **X**) is explained on the last page of this section.

Remember: All pregnancies have a background risk of 3% or more for a serious birth defect, even when mom doesn't take a drug of any kind. If you are pregnant or planning a pregnancy, always let your healthcare provider know before taking any drug, prescription or non-prescription, or herbal remedy.

Rite Aid® Extra Strength Gas Relief Softgels

Active Ingredient:	Pregnancy Risk Category:
Simethicone	C

Helpful Hints and Reminders: Each pregnancy risk category (**A**, **B**, **C**, **D**, or **X**) is explained on the last page of this section.

Remember: All pregnancies have a background risk of 3% or more for a serious birth defect, even when mom doesn't take a drug of any kind. If you are pregnant or planning a pregnancy, always let your healthcare provider know before taking any drug, prescription or non-prescription, or herbal remedy.

Rite Aid® Gas Relief Chewable Tablet Mint Flavor

Active Ingredient:	Pregnancy Risk Category:
Simethicone	C

Helpful Hints and Reminders: Each pregnancy risk category (**A**, **B**, **C**, **D**, or **X**) is explained on the last page of this section.

Remember: All pregnancies have a background risk of 3% or more for a serious birth defect, even when mom doesn't take a drug of any kind. If you are pregnant or planning a pregnancy, always let your healthcare provider know before taking any drug, prescription or non-prescription, or herbal remedy.

Rite Aid® Ultra Strength Gas Relief Softgels

Active Ingredient:	Pregnancy Risk Category:
Simethicone	C

Helpful Hints and Reminders: Each pregnancy risk category (**A**, **B**, **C**, **D**, or **X**) is explained on the last page of this section.

Remember: All pregnancies have a background risk of 3% or more for a serious birth defect, even when mom doesn't take a drug of any kind. If you are pregnant or planning a pregnancy, always let your healthcare provider know before taking any drug, prescription or non-prescription, or herbal remedy.

Rolaids® Extra Strength Plus Gas Relief Soft Chews (Two flavors)

Active Ingredient:	Pregnancy Risk Category:
Calcium carbonate	C
Simethicone	C

Helpful Hints and Reminders: Each pregnancy risk category (**A**, **B**, **C**, **D**, or **X**) is explained on the last page of this section.

Remember: All pregnancies have a background risk of 3% or more for a serious birth defect, even when mom doesn't take a drug of any kind. If you are pregnant or planning a pregnancy, always let your healthcare provider know before taking any drug, prescription or non-prescription, or herbal remedy.

Rolaids® Multi-Symptom Tablets (Two flavors)

Active Ingredient:	Pregnancy Risk Category:
Calcium carbonate	C
Simethicone	C
Magnesium hydroxide	C

Helpful Hints and Reminders: Each pregnancy risk category (**A**, **B**, **C**, **D**, or **X**) is explained on the last page of this section.

Remember: All pregnancies have a background risk of 3% or more for a serious birth defect, even when mom doesn't take a drug of any kind. If you are pregnant or planning a pregnancy, always let your healthcare provider know before taking any drug, prescription or non-prescription, or herbal remedy.

The FDA's Pregnancy Risk Categories: A, B, C, D, X

Adapted to the Active Ingredients in Nonprescription drugs

Category A: Controlled studies using the active ingredient in pregnant women have not shown harmful fetal effects throughout pregnancy, and the possibility of fetal harm seems remote. My comment: *Though apparently safe, these active ingredients should still only be used in pregnancy when clearly indicated.*

Category B: Either studies have shown no evidence of fetal harm when using the active ingredient in pregnant animals, but no controlled studies have been done in pregnant women, **or** studies have shown evidence of fetal harm when using the active ingredient in pregnant animals, but controlled studies in pregnant women have not shown evidence of fetal harm. My comment: *These active ingredients should only be used in pregnancy when clearly indicated.*

Category C: Either studies have shown evidence of fetal harm when using the active ingredient in pregnant animals, but no controlled studies have been done in pregnant women, **or** studies using the active ingredient in pregnant animals have not been done, and studies of pregnant women are insufficient to reach a conclusion. These active ingredients should only be used by a pregnant woman if the potential benefit justifies the potential risk of fetal harm, which, in many cases, is unknown. My comment: *It's impossible to calculate the potential risk of fetal harm when, in many cases, it's unknown. Thus, these active ingredients should only be used in pregnancy when clearly needed.*

Category D: Studies have shown evidence of fetal harm when using the active ingredient in pregnant women. However, the potential benefit of using the active ingredient in some life-threatening situations for

mom may outweigh the potential risk of fetal harm. For example, when mom requires cancer treatment or when she has a serious disease for which safer active ingredients cannot be used or are less effective. My comment: *These exceptional indications rarely occur when considering a nonprescription drug in pregnancy.*

Category X: My comment: *Because the risk of fetal harm is too high, no Category X active ingredients have been approved for use in nonprescription drugs.*

Active Ingredients Assigned Two Pregnancy Risk Categories: Some active ingredients have two pregnancy risk categories, depending on which trimester of pregnancy the active ingredient is used. For example, naproxen sodium, the active ingredient in Aleve, belongs to Category **B** when used in the first and second trimesters of pregnancy. If used in the third trimester, however, the active ingredient belongs to Category **D**. My comment: *This means naproxen sodium should not be used in the third trimester unless prescribed by a physician who has advised her patient of the risks involved.*

Section 7: Heartburn & Reflux Disease

Axid® AR Acid Reducer Tablets

Active Ingredient:	Pregnancy Risk Category:
Nizatidine	B

Helpful Hints and Reminders: Each pregnancy risk category (**A**, **B**, **C**, **D**, or **X**) is explained on the last page of this section.

Remember: All pregnancies have a background risk of 3% or more for a serious birth defect, even when mom doesn't take a drug of any kind. If you are pregnant or planning a pregnancy, always let your healthcare provider know before taking any drug, prescription or non-prescription, or herbal remedy.

CVS® Antacid Liquid Regular Strength Original

Active Ingredient:	Pregnancy Risk Category:
Aluminum hydroxide	C
Magnesium hydroxide	C
Simethicone	C

Helpful Hints and Reminders: Each pregnancy risk category (**A**, **B**, **C**, **D**, or **X**) is explained on the last page of this section.

Remember: All pregnancies have a background risk of 3% or more for a serious birth defect, even when mom doesn't take a drug of any kind. If you are pregnant or planning a pregnancy, always let your healthcare provider know before taking any drug, prescription or non-prescription, or herbal remedy.

CVS® Stomach Relief Caplets

Active Ingredient:	Pregnancy Risk Category:
Bismuth subsalicylate	C (See Helpful Hints below.)

Helpful Hints and Reminders: Each pregnancy risk category (**A**, **B**, **C**, **D**, or **X**) is explained on the last page of this section.

1. "Although the risk of harm may be small, significant adverse fetal effects have resulted from chronic exposure to salicylates. Because of this, the use of bismuth subsalicylate during pregnancy should be restricted to the first half, and then only in amounts that do not exceed the recommended doses," according to G. G. Briggs et al, "Drugs in Pregnancy and Lactation." (See Reference Section in the Appendix.)

Remember: All pregnancies have a background risk of 3% or more for a serious birth defect, even when mom doesn't take a drug of any kind. If you are pregnant or planning a pregnancy, always let your healthcare provider know before taking any drug, prescription or non-prescription, or herbal remedy.

Equate® 75 Mg Acid Reducer

Active Ingredient:	Pregnancy Risk Category:
Ranitidine Hcl	B

Helpful Hints and Reminders: Each pregnancy risk category (**A**, **B**, **C**, **D**, or **X**) is explained on the last page of this section.

Remember: All pregnancies have a background risk of 3% or more for a serious birth defect, even when mom doesn't take a drug of any kind. If you are pregnant or planning a pregnancy, always let your healthcare provider know before taking any drug, prescription or non-prescription, or herbal remedy.

Equate® Antacid Pink-Bismuth Tablets

Active Ingredient:	Pregnancy Risk Category:
Bismuth subsalicylate	**C** (See Helpful Hints below.)

Helpful Hints and Reminders: Each pregnancy risk category (**A**, **B**, **C**, **D**, or **X**) is explained on the last page of this section.

1. "Although the risk of harm may be small, significant adverse fetal effects have resulted from chronic exposure to salicylates. Because of this, the use of bismuth subsalicylate during pregnancy should be restricted to the first half, and then only in amounts that do not exceed the recommended doses," according to G. G. Briggs et al, "Drugs in Pregnancy and Lactation." (See Reference Section in the Appendix.)

Remember: All pregnancies have a background risk of 3% or more for a serious birth defect, even when mom doesn't take a drug of any kind. If you are pregnant or planning a pregnancy, always let your healthcare provider know before taking any drug, prescription or non-prescription, or herbal remedy.

Equate® Chewable Dual Action Acid Reducer Complete Tablets

Active Ingredient:	Pregnancy Risk Category:
Famotidine	**B**
Calcium carbonate	**C**
Magnesium hydroxide	**C**

Helpful Hints and Reminders: Each pregnancy risk category (**A**, **B**, **C**, **D**, or **X**) is explained on the last page of this section.

Remember: All pregnancies have a background risk of 3% or more for a serious birth defect, even when mom doesn't take a drug of any kind. If you are pregnant or planning a pregnancy, always let your healthcare provider know before taking any drug, prescription or non-prescription, or herbal remedy.

Equate® Cimetidine Tablets, 200 Mg Acid Reducer Heartburn Relief

Active Ingredient:	Pregnancy Risk Category:
Cimetidine	B

Helpful Hints and Reminders: Each pregnancy risk category (**A**, **B**, **C**, **D**, or **X**) is explained on the last page of this section.

Remember: All pregnancies have a background risk of 3% or more for a serious birth defect, even when mom doesn't take a drug of any kind. If you are pregnant or planning a pregnancy, always let your healthcare provider know before taking any drug, prescription or non-prescription, or herbal remedy.

Equate® Extra Strength Antacid Tablets

Active Ingredient:	Pregnancy Risk Category:
Aluminum hydroxide	C
Magnesium carbonate	**Risk is undetermined**, but probably small. The FDA has not assigned a pregnancy risk category to this drug. (See Helpful Hints below.)
Simethicone	C

Helpful Hints and Reminders: Each pregnancy risk category (**A**, **B**, **C**, **D**, or **X**) is explained on the last page of this section.

1. There are no controlled studies of magnesium carbonate in pregnancy, like many other drugs. Other magnesium salts, such as magnesium sulfate, have been used extensively during pregnancy in large doses with no reports of birth defects.

Remember: All pregnancies have a background risk of 3% or more for a serious birth defect, even when mom doesn't take a drug of any kind. If you are pregnant or planning a pregnancy, always let your healthcare provider know before taking any drug, prescription or non-prescription, or herbal remedy.

Equate® Extra Strength Assorted Berries Antacid Tablets

Active Ingredient:	Pregnancy Risk Category:
Calcium carbonate	C

Helpful Hints and Reminders: Each pregnancy risk category (**A**, **B**, **C**, **D**, or **X**) is explained on the last page of this section.

Remember: All pregnancies have a background risk of 3% or more for a serious birth defect, even when mom doesn't take a drug of any kind. If you are pregnant or planning a pregnancy, always let your healthcare provider know before taking any drug, prescription or non-prescription, or herbal remedy.

Equate® Liquid Maximum Strength Original Classic Antacid/Anti-Gas

Active Ingredient:	Pregnancy Risk Category:
Aluminum hydroxide	C
Magnesium hydroxide	C
Simethicone	C

Helpful Hints and Reminders: Each pregnancy risk category (**A**, **B**, **C**, **D**, or **X**) is explained on the last page of this section.

Remember: All pregnancies have a background risk of 3% or more for a serious birth defect, even when mom doesn't take a drug of any kind. If you are pregnant or planning a pregnancy, always let your healthcare provider know before taking any drug, prescription or non-prescription, or herbal remedy.

Equate® Maximum Strength Acid Controller & Reducer 20 Mg Tablets

Active Ingredient:	Pregnancy Risk Category:
Famotidine	B

Helpful Hints and Reminders: Each pregnancy risk category (**A**, **B**, **C**, **D**, or **X**) is explained on the last page of this section.

Remember: All pregnancies have a background risk of 3% or more for a serious birth defect, even when mom doesn't take a drug of any kind. If you are pregnant or planning a pregnancy, always let your healthcare provider know before taking any drug, prescription or non-prescription, or herbal remedy.

Equate® Omeprazole Delayed Release Acid Reducer 20 Mg Tablets

Active Ingredient:	Pregnancy Risk Category:
Omeprazole	C

Helpful Hints and Reminders: Each pregnancy risk category (**A**, **B**, **C**, **D**, or **X**) is explained on the last page of this section.

Remember: All pregnancies have a background risk of 3% or more for a serious birth defect, even when mom doesn't take a drug of any kind. If you are pregnant or planning a pregnancy, always let your healthcare provider know before taking any drug, prescription or non-prescription, or herbal remedy.

Equate® Original Effervescent Antacid & Pain Relief

Active Ingredient:	Pregnancy Risk Category:
Citric Acid	**Risk is undetermined.** The FDA has not assigned a pregnancy risk category to this drug.

(continued)

Sodium bicarbonate	C
Aspirin	Aspirin has two pregnancy risk categories: **C** when used in the first or second trimesters of pregnancy; **D** if used in the third trimester. (See Helpful Hints below.)

Helpful Hints and Reminders: Each pregnancy risk category (**A**, **B**, **C**, **D**, or **X**) is explained on the last page of this section.

1. Aspirin is a member of the non-steroidal, anti-inflammatory family of drugs, or NSAIDs. Members of this family of drugs should not be used during the third trimester of pregnancy (last 12 weeks) unless specifically prescribed by a clinician. See the Appendix for "Non-Steroidal, Anti-Inflammatory Drugs (NSAIDs) in Pregnancy," which describes the serious problems these drugs may cause for unborn babies when taken in the third trimester of pregnancy.

2. Women attempting to conceive should not use any NSAID, including aspirin, because of the findings in animals that these drugs may block implantation of the early embryo in the wall of the uterus, in effect preventing pregnancy.

Remember: All pregnancies have a background risk of 3% or more for a serious birth defect, even when mom doesn't take a drug of any kind. If you are pregnant or planning a pregnancy, always let your healthcare provider know before taking any drug, prescription or non-prescription, or herbal remedy.

Equate® Original Strength Acid Controller Famotidine 10 Mg Tablets

Active Ingredient:	Pregnancy Risk Category:
Famotidine	B

Helpful Hints and Reminders: Each pregnancy risk category (**A**, **B**, **C**, **D**, or **X**) is explained on the last page of this section.

Remember: All pregnancies have a background risk of 3% or more for a serious birth defect, even when mom doesn't take a drug of any kind. If you are pregnant or planning a pregnancy, always let your healthcare provider know before taking any drug, prescription or non-prescription, or herbal remedy.

Equate® Regular Strength Liquid Cooling Mint Antacid/Anti-Gas

Active Ingredient:	Pregnancy Risk Category:
Aluminum hydroxide	C
Magnesium hydroxide	C
Simethicone	C

Helpful Hints and Reminders: Each pregnancy risk category (**A**, **B**, **C**, **D**, or **X**) is explained on the last page of this section.

Remember: All pregnancies have a background risk of 3% or more for a serious birth defect, even when mom doesn't take a drug of any kind. If you are pregnant or planning a pregnancy, always let your healthcare provider know before taking any drug, prescription or non-prescription, or herbal remedy.

Equate® Ultra Strength Tropical Fruit Flavors Antacid Tablets

Active Ingredient:	Pregnancy Risk Category:
Calcium carbonate	C

Helpful Hints and Reminders: Each pregnancy risk category (**A**, **B**, **C**, **D**, or **X**) is explained on the last page of this section.

Remember: All pregnancies have a background risk of 3% or more for a serious birth defect, even when mom doesn't take a drug of any kind. If you are pregnant or planning a pregnancy, always let your healthcare provider know before taking any drug, prescription or non-prescription, or herbal remedy.

Gaviscon® Extra Strength Chewable Antacid Tablets

Active Ingredient:	Pregnancy Risk Category:
Aluminum hydroxide	C
Magnesium carbonate	**Risk is undetermined**, but probably small. The FDA has not assigned a pregnancy risk category to this drug. (See Helpful Hints below.)

Helpful Hints and Reminders: Each pregnancy risk category (**A**, **B**, **C**, **D**, or **X**) is explained on the last page of this section.

1. There are no controlled studies of magnesium carbonate in pregnancy, like many other drugs. Other magnesium salts, such as magnesium sulfate, have been used extensively during pregnancy in large doses with no reports of birth defects.

Remember: All pregnancies have a background risk of 3% or more for a serious birth defect, even when mom doesn't take a drug of any kind. If you are pregnant or planning a pregnancy, always let your healthcare provider know before taking any drug, prescription or non-prescription, or herbal remedy.

Gaviscon® Liquid Antacid, Regular Strength, Cool Mint

Active Ingredient:	Pregnancy Risk Category:
Aluminum hydroxide	C
Magnesium carbonate	**Risk is undetermined**, but probably small. The FDA has not assigned a pregnancy risk category to this drug. (See Helpful Hints they are on the next page.)

Kirkland Signature™ Acid Controller Maximum Strength **169**

Helpful Hints and Reminders: Each pregnancy risk category (**A**, **B**, **C**, **D**, or **X**) is explained on the last page of this section.

1. There are no controlled studies of magnesium carbonate in pregnancy, like many other drugs. Other magnesium salts, such as magnesium sulfate, have been used extensively during pregnancy in large doses with no reports of birth defects.

Remember: All pregnancies have a background risk of 3% or more for a serious birth defect, even when mom doesn't take a drug of any kind. If you are pregnant or planning a pregnancy, always let your healthcare provider know before taking any drug, prescription or non-prescription, or herbal remedy.

Gelusil® Antacid/Anti-Gas Tablets

Active Ingredient:	Pregnancy Risk Category:
Aluminum hydroxide	C
Magnesium hydroxide	C
Simethicone	C

Helpful Hints and Reminders: Each pregnancy risk category (**A**, **B**, **C**, **D**, or **X**) is explained on the last page of this section.

Remember: All pregnancies have a background risk of 3% or more for a serious birth defect, even when mom doesn't take a drug of any kind. If you are pregnant or planning a pregnancy, always let your healthcare provider know before taking any drug, prescription or non-prescription, or herbal remedy.

Kirkland Signature™ Acid Controller Maximum Strength

Active Ingredient:	Pregnancy Risk Category:
Famotidine	B

Helpful Hints and Reminders: Each pregnancy risk category (**A**, **B**, **C**, **D**, or **X**) is explained on the last page of this section.

Remember: All pregnancies have a background risk of 3% or more for a serious birth defect, even when mom doesn't take a drug of any kind. If you are pregnant or planning a pregnancy, always let your healthcare provider know before taking any drug, prescription or non-prescription, or herbal remedy.

Kirkland Signature™ Acid Reducer Maximum Strength Ranitidine 150 Mg

Active Ingredient:	Pregnancy Risk Category:
Ranitidine Hcl	**B**

Helpful Hints and Reminders: Each pregnancy risk category (**A**, **B**, **C**, **D**, or **X**) is explained on the last page of this section.

Remember: All pregnancies have a background risk of 3% or more for a serious birth defect, even when mom doesn't take a drug of any kind. If you are pregnant or planning a pregnancy, always let your healthcare provider know before taking any drug, prescription or non-prescription, or herbal remedy.

Kirkland Signature™ Omeprazole Acid Reducer 20 mg Delayed Release

Active Ingredient:	Pregnancy Risk Category:
Omeprazole	**C**

Helpful Hints and Reminders: Each pregnancy risk category (**A**, **B**, **C**, **D**, or **X**) is explained on the last page of this section.

Remember: All pregnancies have a background risk of 3% or more for a serious birth defect, even when mom doesn't take a drug of any kind. If you are pregnant or planning a pregnancy, always let your healthcare provider know before taking any drug, prescription or non-prescription, or herbal remedy.

Maalox® Maximum Strength Multi-Symptom Antacid/Antigas Chewable Tablets

Active Ingredient:	Pregnancy Risk Category:
Calcium carbonate	C
Simethicone	C

Helpful Hints and Reminders: Each pregnancy risk category (**A**, **B**, **C**, **D**, or **X**) is explained on the last page of this section.

Remember: All pregnancies have a background risk of 3% or more for a serious birth defect, even when mom doesn't take a drug of any kind. If you are pregnant or planning a pregnancy, always let your healthcare provider know before taking any drug, prescription or non-prescription, or herbal remedy.

Maalox® Maximum Strength Multi-Symptom Antacid/Antigas Liquid

Active Ingredient:	Pregnancy Risk Category:
Aluminum hydroxide	C
Magnesium hydroxide	C
Simethicone	C

Helpful Hints and Reminders: Each pregnancy risk category (**A**, **B**, **C**, **D**, or **X**) is explained on the last page of this section.

Remember: All pregnancies have a background risk of 3% or more for a serious birth defect, even when mom doesn't take a drug of any kind. If you are pregnant or planning a pregnancy, always let your healthcare provider know before taking any drug, prescription or non-prescription, or herbal remedy.

Maalox® Regular Strength Liquid Antacid & Antigas

Active Ingredient:	Pregnancy Risk Category:
Aluminum hydroxide	C
Magnesium hydroxide	C
Simethicone	C

Helpful Hints and Reminders: Each pregnancy risk category (**A**, **B**, **C**, **D**, or **X**) is explained on the last page of this section.

Remember: All pregnancies have a background risk of 3% or more for a serious birth defect, even when mom doesn't take a drug of any kind. If you are pregnant or planning a pregnancy, always let your healthcare provider know before taking any drug, prescription or non-prescription, or herbal remedy.

Maalox® Total Stomach Relief

Active Ingredient:	Pregnancy Risk Category:
Bismuth subsalicylate	C (See Helpful Hints below.)

Helpful Hints and Reminders: Each pregnancy risk category (**A**, **B**, **C**, **D**, or **X**) is explained on the last page of this section.

1. "Although the risk of harm may be small, significant adverse fetal effects have resulted from chronic exposure to salicylates. Because of this, the use of bismuth subsalicylate during pregnancy should be restricted to the first half, and then only in amounts that do not exceed the recommended doses," according to G. G. Briggs et al, "Drugs in Pregnancy and Lactation." (See Reference Section in the Appendix.)

Remember: All pregnancies have a background risk of 3% or more for a serious birth defect, even when mom doesn't take a drug of any kind. If you are pregnant or planning a pregnancy, always let your healthcare provider know before taking any drug, prescription or non-prescription, or herbal remedy.

Mylanta® Maximum Strength

Active Ingredient:	Pregnancy Risk Category:
Aluminum hydroxide	C
Magnesium hydroxide	C
Simethicone	C

Helpful Hints and Reminders: Each pregnancy risk category (**A**, **B**, **C**, **D**, or **X**) is explained on the last page of this section.

Remember: All pregnancies have a background risk of 3% or more for a serious birth defect, even when mom doesn't take a drug of any kind. If you are pregnant or planning a pregnancy, always let your healthcare provider know before taking any drug, prescription or non-prescription, or herbal remedy.

Mylanta® Regular Strength

Active Ingredient:	Pregnancy Risk Category:
Aluminum hydroxide	C
Magnesium hydroxide	C
Simethicone	C

Helpful Hints and Reminders: Each pregnancy risk category (**A**, **B**, **C**, **D**, or **X**) is explained on the last page of this section.

Remember: All pregnancies have a background risk of 3% or more for a serious birth defect, even when mom doesn't take a drug of any kind. If you are pregnant or planning a pregnancy, always let your healthcare provider know before taking any drug, prescription or non-prescription, or herbal remedy.

Mylanta® Supreme

Active Ingredient:	Pregnancy Risk Category:
Calcium carbonate	C
Magnesium hydroxide	C

Helpful Hints and Reminders: Each pregnancy risk category (**A**, **B**, **C**, **D**, or **X**) is explained on the last page of this section.

Remember: All pregnancies have a background risk of 3% or more for a serious birth defect, even when mom doesn't take a drug of any kind. If you are pregnant or planning a pregnancy, always let your healthcare provider know before taking any drug, prescription or non-prescription, or herbal remedy.

Mylanta® Ultimate Strength Chewables

Active Ingredient:	Pregnancy Risk Category:
Calcium carbonate	C
Magnesium hydroxide	C

Helpful Hints and Reminders: Each pregnancy risk category (**A**, **B**, **C**, **D**, or **X**) is explained on the last page of this section.

Remember: All pregnancies have a background risk of 3% or more for a serious birth defect, even when mom doesn't take a drug of any kind. If you are pregnant or planning a pregnancy, always let your healthcare provider know before taking any drug, prescription or non-prescription, or herbal remedy.

Mylanta® Ultimate Strength Liquid

Active Ingredient:	Pregnancy Risk Category:
Aluminum hydroxide	C
Magnesium hydroxide	C

Helpful Hints and Reminders: Each pregnancy risk category (**A**, **B**, **C**, **D**, or **X**) is explained on the last page of this section.

Remember: All pregnancies have a background risk of 3% or more for a serious birth defect, even when mom doesn't take a drug of any kind. If you are pregnant or planning a pregnancy, always let your healthcare provider know before taking any drug, prescription or non-prescription, or herbal remedy.

Pepcid® AC® Maximum Strength Tablets & EZ Chews

Active Ingredient:	Pregnancy Risk Category:
Famotidine	B

Helpful Hints and Reminders: Each pregnancy risk category (**A**, **B**, **C**, **D**, or **X**) is explained on the last page of this section.

Remember: All pregnancies have a background risk of 3% or more for a serious birth defect, even when mom doesn't take a drug of any kind. If you are pregnant or planning a pregnancy, always let your healthcare provider know before taking any drug, prescription or non-prescription, or herbal remedy.

Pepcid® AC® Original Strength, Gelcaps & Tablets

Active Ingredient:	Pregnancy Risk Category:
Famotidine	B

Helpful Hints and Reminders: Each pregnancy risk category (**A**, **B**, **C**, **D**, or **X**) is explained on the last page of this section.

Remember: All pregnancies have a background risk of 3% or more for a serious birth defect, even when mom doesn't take a drug of any kind. If you are pregnant or planning a pregnancy, always let your healthcare provider know before taking any drug, prescription or non-prescription, or herbal remedy.

Pepcid® Complete®, Chewable Tablets Three Flavors

Active Ingredient:	Pregnancy Risk Category:
Famotidine	B
Calcium carbonate	C
Magnesium hydroxide	C

Helpful Hints and Reminders: Each pregnancy risk category (**A**, **B**, **C**, **D**, or **X**) is explained on the last page of this section.

Remember: All pregnancies have a background risk of 3% or more for a serious birth defect, even when mom doesn't take a drug of any kind. If you are pregnant or planning a pregnancy, always let your healthcare provider know before taking any drug, prescription or non-prescription, or herbal remedy.

Pepto-Bismol®, Original & Maximum Strength

Active Ingredient:	Pregnancy Risk Category:
Bismuth subsalicylate	C (See Helpful Hints below.)

Helpful Hints and Reminders: Each pregnancy risk category (**A**, **B**, **C**, **D**, or **X**) is explained on the last page of this section.

1. "Although the risk of harm may be small, significant adverse fetal effects have resulted from chronic exposure to salicylates. Because of this, the use of bismuth subsalicylate during pregnancy should be restricted to the first half, and then only in amounts that do not exceed the recommended doses," according to G. G. Briggs et al, "Drugs in Pregnancy and Lactation." (See Reference Section in the Appendix.)

Remember: All pregnancies have a background risk of 3% or more for a serious birth defect, even when mom doesn't take a drug of any kind. If you are pregnant or planning a pregnancy, always let your healthcare provider know before taking any drug, prescription or non-prescription, or herbal remedy.

Phillips® Genuine Milk of Magnesia

Active Ingredient:	Pregnancy Risk Category:
Magnesium hydroxide	C

Helpful Hints and Reminders: Each pregnancy risk category (**A**, **B**, **C**, **D**, or **X**) is explained on the last page of this section.

Remember: All pregnancies have a background risk of 3% or more for a serious birth defect, even when mom doesn't take a drug of any kind. If you are pregnant or planning a pregnancy, always let your healthcare provider know before taking any drug, prescription or non-prescription, or herbal remedy.

Prilosec OTC® Tablets

Active Ingredient:	Pregnancy Risk Category:
Omeprazole	C

Helpful Hints and Reminders: Each pregnancy risk category (**A**, **B**, **C**, **D**, or **X**) is explained on the last page of this section.

Remember: All pregnancies have a background risk of 3% or more for a serious birth defect, even when mom doesn't take a drug of any kind. If you are pregnant or planning a pregnancy, always let your healthcare provider know before taking any drug, prescription or non-prescription, or herbal remedy.

Rite Aid® Antacid & Anti-Gas Original

Active Ingredient:	Pregnancy Risk Category:
Aluminum hydroxide	C
Magnesium hydroxide	C
Simethicone	C

Helpful Hints and Reminders: Each pregnancy risk category (**A**, **B**, **C**, **D**, or **X**) is explained on the last page of this section.

Remember: All pregnancies have a background risk of 3% or more for a serious birth defect, even when mom doesn't take a drug of any kind. If you are pregnant or planning a pregnancy, always let your healthcare provider know before taking any drug, prescription or non-prescription, or herbal remedy.

Rolaids® Extra Strength Plus Gas Relief Soft Chews (Two flavors)

Active Ingredient:	Pregnancy Risk Category:
Calcium carbonate	C
Simethicone	C

Helpful Hints and Reminders: Each pregnancy risk category (**A**, **B**, **C**, **D**, or **X**) is explained on the last page of this section.

Remember: All pregnancies have a background risk of 3% or more for a serious birth defect, even when mom doesn't take a drug of any kind. If you are pregnant or planning a pregnancy, always let your healthcare provider know before taking any drug, prescription or non-prescription, or herbal remedy.

Rolaids® Extra Strength Softchews

Active Ingredient:	Pregnancy Risk Category:
Calcium carbonate	C

Helpful Hints and Reminders: Each pregnancy risk category (**A**, **B**, **C**, **D**, or **X**) is explained on the last page of this section.

Remember: All pregnancies have a background risk of 3% or more for a serious birth defect, even when mom doesn't take a drug of any kind. If you are pregnant or planning a pregnancy, always let your healthcare provider know before taking any drug, prescription or non-prescription, or herbal remedy.

Rolaids® Extra Strength Tablets (Three flavors)

Active Ingredient:	Pregnancy Risk Category:
Calcium carbonate	C
Magnesium hydroxide	C

Helpful Hints and Reminders: Each pregnancy risk category (**A**, **B**, **C**, **D**, or **X**) is explained on the last page of this section.

Remember: All pregnancies have a background risk of 3% or more for a serious birth defect, even when mom doesn't take a drug of any kind. If you are pregnant or planning a pregnancy, always let your healthcare provider know before taking any drug, prescription or non-prescription, or herbal remedy.

Rolaids® Multi-Symptom Tablets (Two flavors)

Active Ingredient:	Pregnancy Risk Category:
Calcium carbonate	C
Simethicone	C
Magnesium hydroxide	C

Helpful Hints and Reminders: Each pregnancy risk category (**A**, **B**, **C**, **D**, or **X**) is explained on the last page of this section.

Remember: All pregnancies have a background risk of 3% or more for a serious birth defect, even when mom doesn't take a drug of any kind. If you are pregnant or planning a pregnancy, always let your healthcare provider know before taking any drug, prescription or non-prescription, or herbal remedy.

Rolaids® Regular Strength Tablets (Two flavors)

Active Ingredient:	Pregnancy Risk Category:
Calcium carbonate	C
Magnesium hydroxide	C

Helpful Hints and Reminders: Each pregnancy risk category (**A**, **B**, **C**, **D**, or **X**) is explained on the last page of this section.

Remember: All pregnancies have a background risk of 3% or more for a serious birth defect, even when mom doesn't take a drug of any kind. If you are pregnant or planning a pregnancy, always let your healthcare

provider know before taking any drug, prescription or non-prescription, or herbal remedy.

Target® Antacid Anti-Gas Liquid

Active Ingredient:	Pregnancy Risk Category:
Magnesium hydroxide	C
Aluminum hydroxide	C
Simethicone	C

Helpful Hints and Reminders: Each pregnancy risk category (**A**, **B**, **C**, **D**, or **X**) is explained on the last page of this section.

Remember: All pregnancies have a background risk of 3% or more for a serious birth defect, even when mom doesn't take a drug of any kind. If you are pregnant or planning a pregnancy, always let your healthcare provider know before taking any drug, prescription or non-prescription, or herbal remedy.

Target® Famotidine Acid Reducer Complete Mint Chews

Active Ingredient:	Pregnancy Risk Category:
Famotidine	B
Magnesium hydroxide	C
Calcium carbonate	C

Helpful Hints and Reminders: Each pregnancy risk category (**A**, **B**, **C**, **D**, or **X**) is explained on the last page of this section.

Remember: All pregnancies have a background risk of 3% or more for a serious birth defect, even when mom doesn't take a drug of any kind. If you are pregnant or planning a pregnancy, always let your healthcare provider know before taking any drug, prescription or non-prescription, or herbal remedy.

Target® Famotidine Acid Relief Tablets

Active Ingredient:	Pregnancy Risk Category:
Famotidine	B

Helpful Hints and Reminders: Each pregnancy risk category (**A**, **B**, **C**, **D**, or **X**) is explained on the last page of this section.

Remember: All pregnancies have a background risk of 3% or more for a serious birth defect, even when mom doesn't take a drug of any kind. If you are pregnant or planning a pregnancy, always let your healthcare provider know before taking any drug, prescription or non-prescription, or herbal remedy.

Target® Omeprazole 20 Mg Acid Relief Tablets

Active Ingredient:	Pregnancy Risk Category:
Omeprazole	C

Helpful Hints and Reminders: Each pregnancy risk category (**A**, **B**, **C**, **D**, or **X**) is explained on the last page of this section.

Remember: All pregnancies have a background risk of 3% or more for a serious birth defect, even when mom doesn't take a drug of any kind. If you are pregnant or planning a pregnancy, always let your healthcare provider know before taking any drug, prescription or non-prescription, or herbal remedy.

Target® Ranitidine Acid Relief Tablets

Active Ingredient:	Pregnancy Risk Category:
Ranitidine	B

Helpful Hints and Reminders: Each pregnancy risk category (**A**, **B**, **C**, **D**, or **X**) is explained on the last page of this section.

Remember: All pregnancies have a background risk of 3% or more for a serious birth defect, even when mom doesn't take a drug of any kind. If you are pregnant or planning a pregnancy, always let your healthcare

provider know before taking any drug, prescription or non-prescription, or herbal remedy.

Tums® E-X 750 (Four flavors)

Active Ingredient:	Pregnancy Risk Category:
Calcium carbonate	C

Helpful Hints and Reminders: Each pregnancy risk category (**A**, **B**, **C**, **D**, or **X**) is explained on the last page of this section.

Remember: All pregnancies have a background risk of 3% or more for a serious birth defect, even when mom doesn't take a drug of any kind. If you are pregnant or planning a pregnancy, always let your healthcare provider know before taking any drug, prescription or non-prescription, or herbal remedy.

Tums® E-X Sugar Free

Active Ingredient:	Pregnancy Risk Category:
Calcium carbonate	C

Helpful Hints and Reminders: Each pregnancy risk category (**A**, **B**, **C**, **D**, or **X**) is explained on the last page of this section.

Remember: All pregnancies have a background risk of 3% or more for a serious birth defect, even when mom doesn't take a drug of any kind. If you are pregnant or planning a pregnancy, always let your healthcare provider know before taking any drug, prescription or non-prescription, or herbal remedy.

Tums® New Dual Action (Two flavors)

Active Ingredient:	Pregnancy Risk Category:
Calcium carbonate	C
Famotidine	B
Magnesium hydroxide	C

Helpful Hints and Reminders: Each pregnancy risk category (**A**, **B**, **C**, **D**, or **X**) is explained on the last page of this section.

Remember: All pregnancies have a background risk of 3% or more for a serious birth defect, even when mom doesn't take a drug of any kind. If you are pregnant or planning a pregnancy, always let your healthcare provider know before taking any drug, prescription or non-prescription, or herbal remedy.

Tums® New Quik Pak

Active Ingredient:	Pregnancy Risk Category:
Calcium carbonate	C

Helpful Hints and Reminders: Each pregnancy risk category (**A**, **B**, **C**, **D**, or **X**) is explained on the last page of this section.

Remember: All pregnancies have a background risk of 3% or more for a serious birth defect, even when mom doesn't take a drug of any kind. If you are pregnant or planning a pregnancy, always let your healthcare provider know before taking any drug, prescription or non-prescription, or herbal remedy.

Tums® Regular Strength (Two flavors)

Active Ingredient:	Pregnancy Risk Category:
Calcium carbonate	C

Helpful Hints and Reminders: Each pregnancy risk category (**A**, **B**, **C**, **D**, or **X**) is explained on the last page of this section.

Remember: All pregnancies have a background risk of 3% or more for a serious birth defect, even when mom doesn't take a drug of any kind. If you are pregnant or planning a pregnancy, always let your healthcare provider know before taking any drug, prescription or non-prescription, or herbal remedy.

Tums® Smoothies (Five flavors)

Active Ingredient:	Pregnancy Risk Category:
Calcium carbonate	C

Helpful Hints and Reminders: Each pregnancy risk category (**A**, **B**, **C**, **D**, or **X**) is explained on the last page of this section.

Remember: All pregnancies have a background risk of 3% or more for a serious birth defect, even when mom doesn't take a drug of any kind. If you are pregnant or planning a pregnancy, always let your healthcare provider know before taking any drug, prescription or non-prescription, or herbal remedy.

Tums® Ultra 1000 (Four flavors)

Active Ingredient:	Pregnancy Risk Category:
Calcium carbonate	C

Helpful Hints and Reminders: Each pregnancy risk category (**A**, **B**, **C**, **D**, or **X**) is explained on the last page of this section.

Remember: All pregnancies have a background risk of 3% or more for a serious birth defect, even when mom doesn't take a drug of any kind. If you are pregnant or planning a pregnancy, always let your healthcare provider know before taking any drug, prescription or non-prescription, or herbal remedy.

Walgreens® Assorted Fruit Extra 750 mg Antacid Chewable Tablets

Active Ingredient:	Pregnancy Risk Category:
Calcium carbonate	C

Helpful Hints and Reminders: Each pregnancy risk category (**A**, **B**, **C**, **D**, or **X**) is explained on the last page of this section.

Remember: All pregnancies have a background risk of 3% or more for a serious birth defect, even when mom doesn't take a drug of any kind.

If you are pregnant or planning a pregnancy, always let your healthcare provider know before taking any drug, prescription or non-prescription, or herbal remedy.

Walgreens® Extra Strength Antacid Tablets

Active Ingredient:	Pregnancy Risk Category:
Calcium carbonate	C

Helpful Hints and Reminders: Each pregnancy risk category (**A**, **B**, **C**, **D**, or **X**) is explained on the last page of this section.

Remember: All pregnancies have a background risk of 3% or more for a serious birth defect, even when mom doesn't take a drug of any kind. If you are pregnant or planning a pregnancy, always let your healthcare provider know before taking any drug, prescription or non-prescription, or herbal remedy.

Walgreens® Maximum Strength Acid Controller Tablets

Active Ingredient:	Pregnancy Risk Category:
Famotidine	B

Helpful Hints and Reminders: Each pregnancy risk category (**A**, **B**, **C**, **D**, or **X**) is explained on the last page of this section.

Remember: All pregnancies have a background risk of 3% or more for a serious birth defect, even when mom doesn't take a drug of any kind. If you are pregnant or planning a pregnancy, always let your healthcare provider know before taking any drug, prescription or non-prescription, or herbal remedy.

Walgreens® Omeprazole Acid Reducer

Active Ingredient:	Pregnancy Risk Category:
Omeprazole	C

Helpful Hints and Reminders: Each pregnancy risk category (**A**, **B**, **C**, **D**, or **X**) is explained on the last page of this section.

Remember: All pregnancies have a background risk of 3% or more for a serious birth defect, even when mom doesn't take a drug of any kind. If you are pregnant or planning a pregnancy, always let your healthcare provider know before taking any drug, prescription or non-prescription, or herbal remedy.

Zantac® Ranitidine Tablets 75 Mg Acid Reducer

Active Ingredient:	Pregnancy Risk Category:
Ranitidine	B

Helpful Hints and Reminders: Each pregnancy risk category (**A**, **B**, **C**, **D**, or **X**) is explained on the last page of this section.

Remember: All pregnancies have a background risk of 3% or more for a serious birth defect, even when mom doesn't take a drug of any kind. If you are pregnant or planning a pregnancy, always let your healthcare provider know before taking any drug, prescription or non-prescription, or herbal remedy.

Zantac® Ranitidine Tablets 150 Mg Maximum Strength Acid Reducer

Active Ingredient:	Pregnancy Risk Category:
Ranitidine	B

Helpful Hints and Reminders: Each pregnancy risk category (**A**, **B**, **C**, **D**, or **X**) is explained on the last page of this section.

Remember: All pregnancies have a background risk of 3% or more for a serious birth defect, even when mom doesn't take a drug of any kind. If you are pregnant or planning a pregnancy, always let your healthcare provider know before taking any drug, prescription or non-prescription, or herbal remedy.

Zegerid OTC Capsules

Active Ingredient:	Pregnancy Risk Category:
Omeprazole	C
Sodium bicarbonate	C

Helpful Hints and Reminders: Each pregnancy risk category (**A**, **B**, **C**, **D**, or **X**) is explained on the last page of this section.

Remember: All pregnancies have a background risk of 3% or more for a serious birth defect, even when mom doesn't take a drug of any kind. If you are pregnant or planning a pregnancy, always let your healthcare provider know before taking any drug, prescription or non-prescription, or herbal remedy.

The FDA's Pregnancy Risk Categories: A, B, C, D, X

Adapted to the Active Ingredients in Nonprescription drugs

Category A: Controlled studies using the active ingredient in pregnant women have not shown harmful fetal effects throughout pregnancy, and the possibility of fetal harm seems remote. My comment: *Though apparently safe, these active ingredients should still only be used in pregnancy when clearly indicated.*

Category B: Either studies have shown no evidence of fetal harm when using the active ingredient in pregnant animals, but no controlled studies have been done in pregnant women, **or** studies have shown evidence of fetal harm when using the active ingredient in pregnant animals, but controlled studies in pregnant women have not shown evidence of fetal harm. My comment: *These active ingredients should only be used in pregnancy when clearly indicated.*

Category C: Either studies have shown evidence of fetal harm when using the active ingredient in pregnant animals, but no controlled studies have been done in pregnant women, **or** studies using the active ingredient in pregnant animals have not been done, and studies of pregnant women are insufficient to reach a conclusion. These active ingredients should only be used by a pregnant woman if the potential benefit justifies the potential risk of fetal harm, which, in many cases, is unknown. My comment: *It's impossible to calculate the potential risk of fetal harm when, in many cases, it's unknown. Thus, these active ingredients should only be used in pregnancy when clearly needed.*

Category D: Studies have shown evidence of fetal harm when using the active ingredient in pregnant women. However, the potential benefit of using the active ingredient in some life-threatening situations for

mom may outweigh the potential risk of fetal harm. For example, when mom requires cancer treatment or when she has a serious disease for which safer active ingredients cannot be used or are less effective. My comment: *These exceptional indications rarely occur when considering a nonprescription drug in pregnancy.*

Category X: My comment: *Because the risk of fetal harm is too high, no Category X active ingredients have been approved for use in nonprescription drugs.*

Active Ingredients Assigned Two Pregnancy Risk Categories: Some active ingredients have two pregnancy risk categories, depending on which trimester of pregnancy the active ingredient is used. For example, naproxen sodium, the active ingredient in Aleve, belongs to Category **B** when used in the first and second trimesters of pregnancy. If used in the third trimester, however, the active ingredient belongs to Category **D**. My comment: *This means naproxen sodium should not be used in the third trimester unless prescribed by a physician who has advised her patient of the risks involved.*

Section 8: Menstrual Discomfort

CVS® Menstrual Relief, Menstrual Complete Gelcaps or Caplets

Active Ingredient:	Pregnancy Risk Category:
Acetaminophen	B
Pyrilamine maleate	C
Caffeine	B

Helpful Hints and Reminders: Each pregnancy risk category (**A**, **B**, **C**, **D**, or **X**) is explained on the last page of this section.

Remember: All pregnancies have a background risk of 3% or more for a serious birth defect, even when mom doesn't take a drug of any kind. If you are pregnant or planning a pregnancy, always let your healthcare provider know before taking any drug, prescription or non-prescription, or herbal remedy.

Excedrin® Menstrual Complete Express Gels

Active Ingredient:	Pregnancy Risk Category:
Acetaminophen	B
Caffeine	B

(continued)

| Aspirin | Aspirin has two pregnancy risk categories: **C** when used in the first or second trimesters of pregnancy; **D** if used in the third trimester. (See Helpful Hints below.) |

Helpful Hints and Reminders: Each pregnancy risk category (**A**, **B**, **C**, **D**, or **X**) is explained on the last page of this section.

1. Aspirin is a member of the non-steroidal, anti-inflammatory family of drugs, or NSAIDs. Members of this family of drugs should not be used during the third trimester of pregnancy (last 12 weeks) unless specifically prescribed by a clinician. See the Appendix for "Non-Steroidal, Anti-Inflammatory Drugs (NSAIDs) in Pregnancy," which describes the serious problems these drugs may cause for unborn babies when taken in the third trimester of pregnancy.

2. Women attempting to conceive should not use any NSAID, including aspirin, because of the findings in animals that these drugs may block implantation of the early embryo in the wall of the uterus, in effect preventing pregnancy.

Remember: All pregnancies have a background risk of 3% or more for a serious birth defect, even when mom doesn't take a drug of any kind. If you are pregnant or planning a pregnancy, always let your healthcare provider know before taking any drug, prescription or non-prescription, or herbal remedy.

Midol® Complete

Active Ingredient:	Pregnancy Risk Category:
Acetaminophen	B
Caffeine	B
Pyrilamine maleate	C

Helpful Hints and Reminders: Each pregnancy risk category (**A**, **B**, **C**, **D**, or **X**) is explained on the last page of this section.

Remember: All pregnancies have a background risk of 3% or more for a serious birth defect, even when mom doesn't take a drug of any kind. If you are pregnant or planning a pregnancy, always let your healthcare provider know before taking any drug, prescription or non-prescription, or herbal remedy.

Midol® Extended Relief

Active Ingredient:	Pregnancy Risk Category:
Naproxen sodium	Naproxen sodium has two pregnancy risk categories: **C** when used in the first or second trimesters of pregnancy; **D** if used in the third trimester. (See Helpful Hints below.)

Helpful Hints and Reminders: Each pregnancy risk category (**A**, **B**, **C**, **D**, or **X**) is explained on the last page of this section.

1. Naproxen sodium is a member of the non-steroidal, anti-inflammatory family of drugs, or NSAIDs. Members of this family of drugs should not be used during the third trimester of pregnancy (last 12 weeks) unless specifically prescribed by a clinician. See the Appendix for "Non-Steroidal, Anti-Inflammatory Drugs (NSAIDs) in Pregnancy," which describes the serious problems these drugs may cause for unborn babies when taken in the third trimester of pregnancy.

2. Women attempting to conceive should not use any NSAID, including naproxen sodium, because of the findings in animals that these drugs may block implantation of the early embryo in the wall of the uterus, in effect preventing pregnancy.

Remember: All pregnancies have a background risk of 3% or more for a serious birth defect, even when mom doesn't take a drug of any kind. If you are pregnant or planning a pregnancy, always let your healthcare provider know before taking any drug, prescription or non-prescription, or herbal remedy.

Midol® Liquid Gels

Active Ingredient:	Pregnancy Risk Category:
Ibuprofen	Ibuprofen has two pregnancy risk categories: **B** when used in the first or second trimesters of pregnancy; **D** if used in the third trimester. (See Helpful Hints below.)

Helpful Hints and Reminders: Each pregnancy risk category (**A**, **B**, **C**, **D**, or **X**) is explained on the last page of this section.

1. Ibuprofen is a member of the non-steroidal, anti-inflammatory family of drugs, or NSAIDs. Members of this family of drugs should not be used during the third trimester of pregnancy (last 12 weeks) unless specifically prescribed by a clinician. See the Appendix for "Non-Steroidal, Anti-Inflammatory Drugs (NSAIDs) in Pregnancy," which describes the serious problems these drugs may cause for unborn babies when taken in the third trimester of pregnancy.

2. Women attempting to conceive should not use any NSAID, including ibuprofen, because of the findings in animals that these drugs may block implantation of the early embryo in the wall of the uterus, in effect preventing pregnancy.

Remember: All pregnancies have a background risk of 3% or more for a serious birth defect, even when mom doesn't take a drug of any kind. If you are pregnant or planning a pregnancy, always let your healthcare provider know before taking any drug, prescription or non-prescription, or herbal remedy.

Midol® PM

Active Ingredient:	Pregnancy Risk Category:
Acetaminophen	B
Diphenhydramine citrate	B

Helpful Hints and Reminders: Each pregnancy risk category (**A**, **B**, **C**, **D**, or **X**) is explained on the last page of this section.

Remember: All pregnancies have a background risk of 3% or more for a serious birth defect, even when mom doesn't take a drug of any kind. If you are pregnant or planning a pregnancy, always let your healthcare provider know before taking any drug, prescription or non-prescription, or herbal remedy.

Midol® Teen Formula

Active Ingredient:	Pregnancy Risk Category:
Acetaminophen	B
Pamabrom	**Risk is undetermined.** The FDA has not assigned this drug to a pregnancy risk category. Clinical experience suggests fetal risk from exposure during pregnancy is low, according to some experts.

Helpful Hints and Reminders: Each pregnancy risk category (**A**, **B**, **C**, **D**, or **X**) is explained on the last page of this section.

Remember: All pregnancies have a background risk of 3% or more for a serious birth defect, even when mom doesn't take a drug of any kind. If you are pregnant or planning a pregnancy, always let your healthcare provider know before taking any drug, prescription or non-prescription, or herbal remedy.

Walgreens® Menstrual Relief Aspirin Free Caplets Maximum Strength

Active Ingredient:	Pregnancy Risk Category:
Acetaminophen	B
Caffeine	B
Pyrilamine maleate	C

Walgreens® Menstrual Relief Aspirin Free Caplets Maximum Strength **195**

Helpful Hints and Reminders: Each pregnancy risk category (**A**, **B**, **C**, **D**, or **X**) is explained on the last page of this section.

Remember: All pregnancies have a background risk of 3% or more for a serious birth defect, even when mom doesn't take a drug of any kind. If you are pregnant or planning a pregnancy, always let your healthcare provider know before taking any drug, prescription or non-prescription, or herbal remedy.

The FDA's Pregnancy Risk Categories: A, B, C, D, X

Adapted to the Active Ingredients in Nonprescription drugs

Category A: Controlled studies using the active ingredient in pregnant women have not shown harmful fetal effects throughout pregnancy, and the possibility of fetal harm seems remote. My comment: *Though apparently safe, these active ingredients should still only be used in pregnancy when clearly indicated.*

Category B: Either studies have shown no evidence of fetal harm when using the active ingredient in pregnant animals, but no controlled studies have been done in pregnant women, **or** studies have shown evidence of fetal harm when using the active ingredient in pregnant animals, but controlled studies in pregnant women have not shown evidence of fetal harm. My comment: *These active ingredients should only be used in pregnancy when clearly indicated.*

Category C: Either studies have shown evidence of fetal harm when using the active ingredient in pregnant animals, but no controlled studies have been done in pregnant women, **or** studies using the active ingredient in pregnant animals have not been done, and studies of pregnant women are insufficient to reach a conclusion. These active ingredients should only be used by a pregnant woman if the potential benefit justifies the potential risk of fetal harm, which, in many cases, is unknown. My comment: *It's impossible to calculate the potential risk of fetal harm when, in many cases, it's unknown. Thus, these active ingredients should only be used in pregnancy when clearly needed.*

Category D: Studies have shown evidence of fetal harm when using the active ingredient in pregnant women. However, the potential benefit of using the active ingredient in some life-threatening situations for

mom may outweigh the potential risk of fetal harm. For example, when mom requires cancer treatment or when she has a serious disease for which safer active ingredients cannot be used or are less effective. My comment: *These exceptional indications rarely occur when considering a nonprescription drug in pregnancy.*

Category X: My comment: *Because the risk of fetal harm is too high, no Category X active ingredients have been approved for use in nonprescription drugs.*

Active Ingredients Assigned Two Pregnancy Risk Categories: Some active ingredients have two pregnancy risk categories, depending on which trimester of pregnancy the active ingredient is used. For example, naproxen sodium, the active ingredient in Aleve, belongs to Category **B** when used in the first and second trimesters of pregnancy. If used in the third trimester, however, the active ingredient belongs to Category **D**. My comment: *This means naproxen sodium should not be used in the third trimester unless prescribed by a physician who has advised her patient of the risks involved.*

Section 9: Motion Sickness

Bonine® Motion Sickness Protection, Raspberry Chewable Tablets

Active Ingredient:	Pregnancy Risk Category:
Meclizine Hcl	B

Helpful Hints and Reminders: Each pregnancy risk category (**A**, **B**, **C**, **D**, or **X**) is explained on the last page of this section.

Remember: All pregnancies have a background risk of 3% or more for a serious birth defect, even when mom doesn't take a drug of any kind. If you are pregnant or planning a pregnancy, always let your healthcare provider know before taking any drug, prescription or non-prescription, or herbal remedy.

CVS® Motion Sickness II Tablets Less Drowsy Formula

Active Ingredient:	Pregnancy Risk Category:
Meclizine Hcl	B

Helpful Hints and Reminders: Each pregnancy risk category (**A**, **B**, **C**, **D**, or **X**) is explained on the last page of this section.

Remember: All pregnancies have a background risk of 3% or more for a serious birth defect, even when mom doesn't take a drug of any kind.

Dramamine® Chewable Tablets

If you are pregnant or planning a pregnancy, always let your healthcare provider know before taking any drug, prescription or non-prescription, or herbal remedy.

CVS® Motion Sickness Relief Raspberry Flavored Tablet

Active Ingredient:	Pregnancy Risk Category:
Meclizine Hcl	B

Helpful Hints and Reminders: Each pregnancy risk category (**A**, **B**, **C**, **D**, or **X**) is explained on the last page of this section.

Remember: All pregnancies have a background risk of 3% or more for a serious birth defect, even when mom doesn't take a drug of any kind. If you are pregnant or planning a pregnancy, always let your healthcare provider know before taking any drug, prescription or non-prescription, or herbal remedy.

CVS® Motion Sickness Tablets Original Formula

Active Ingredient:	Pregnancy Risk Category:
Dimenhydrinate	B

Helpful Hints and Reminders: Each pregnancy risk category (**A**, **B**, **C**, **D**, or **X**) is explained on the last page of this section.

Remember: All pregnancies have a background risk of 3% or more for a serious birth defect, even when mom doesn't take a drug of any kind. If you are pregnant or planning a pregnancy, always let your healthcare provider know before taking any drug, prescription or non-prescription, or herbal remedy.

Dramamine® Chewable Tablets

Active Ingredient:	Pregnancy Risk Category:
Dimenhydrinate	B

Helpful Hints and Reminders: Each pregnancy risk category (**A**, **B**, **C**, **D**, or **X**) is explained on the last page of this section.

Remember: All pregnancies have a background risk of 3% or more for a serious birth defect, even when mom doesn't take a drug of any kind. If you are pregnant or planning a pregnancy, always let your healthcare provider know before taking any drug, prescription or non-prescription, or herbal remedy.

Dramamine® Less Drowsy Formula

Active Ingredient:	Pregnancy Risk Category:
Meclizine Hcl	B

Helpful Hints and Reminders: Each pregnancy risk category (**A**, **B**, **C**, **D**, or **X**) is explained on the last page of this section.

Remember: All pregnancies have a background risk of 3% or more for a serious birth defect, even when mom doesn't take a drug of any kind. If you are pregnant or planning a pregnancy, always let your healthcare provider know before taking any drug, prescription or non-prescription, or herbal remedy.

Dramamine® Original Formula

Active Ingredient:	Pregnancy Risk Category:
Dimenhydrinate	B

Helpful Hints and Reminders: Each pregnancy risk category (**A**, **B**, **C**, **D**, or **X**) is explained on the last page of this section.

Remember: All pregnancies have a background risk of 3% or more for a serious birth defect, even when mom doesn't take a drug of any kind. If you are pregnant or planning a pregnancy, always let your healthcare provider know before taking any drug, prescription or non-prescription, or herbal remedy.

Equate® Motion Sickness Tablets

Active Ingredient:	Pregnancy Risk Category:
Dimenhydrinate	B

Meclizine HCL, USP 25 Mg Antiemetic Tablets **201**

Helpful Hints and Reminders: Each pregnancy risk category (**A**, **B**, **C**, **D**, or **X**) is explained on the last page of this section.

Remember: All pregnancies have a background risk of 3% or more for a serious birth defect, even when mom doesn't take a drug of any kind. If you are pregnant or planning a pregnancy, always let your healthcare provider know before taking any drug, prescription or non-prescription, or herbal remedy.

Marezine® 50 Mg Motion Sickness Tablets

Active Ingredient:	Pregnancy Risk Category:
Cyclizine Hcl	B

Helpful Hints and Reminders: Each pregnancy risk category (**A**, **B**, **C**, **D**, or **X**) is explained on the last page of this section.

Remember: All pregnancies have a background risk of 3% or more for a serious birth defect, even when mom doesn't take a drug of any kind. If you are pregnant or planning a pregnancy, always let your healthcare provider know before taking any drug, prescription or non-prescription, or herbal remedy.

Meclizine HCL, USP 25 Mg Antiemetic Tablets

Active Ingredient:	Pregnancy Risk Category:
Meclizine Hcl	B

Helpful Hints and Reminders: Each pregnancy risk category (**A**, **B**, **C**, **D**, or **X**) is explained on the last page of this section.

Remember: All pregnancies have a background risk of 3% or more for a serious birth defect, even when mom doesn't take a drug of any kind. If you are pregnant or planning a pregnancy, always let your healthcare provider know before taking any drug, prescription or non-prescription, or herbal remedy.

Rite Aid® Motion Sickness Relief Tablets

Active Ingredient:	Pregnancy Risk Category:
Dimenhydrinate	B

Helpful Hints and Reminders: Each pregnancy risk category (**A**, **B**, **C**, **D**, or **X**) is explained on the last page of this section.

Remember: All pregnancies have a background risk of 3% or more for a serious birth defect, even when mom doesn't take a drug of any kind. If you are pregnant or planning a pregnancy, always let your healthcare provider know before taking any drug, prescription or non-prescription, or herbal remedy.

Rugby® Travel Sickness Tablets

Active Ingredient:	Pregnancy Risk Category:
Meclizine Hcl	B

Helpful Hints and Reminders: Each pregnancy risk category (**A**, **B**, **C**, **D**, or **X**) is explained on the last page of this section.

Remember: All pregnancies have a background risk of 3% or more for a serious birth defect, even when mom doesn't take a drug of any kind. If you are pregnant or planning a pregnancy, always let your healthcare provider know before taking any drug, prescription or non-prescription, or herbal remedy.

Triptone® For Motion Sickness Tablets

Active Ingredient:	Pregnancy Risk Category:
Dimenhydrinate	B

Helpful Hints and Reminders: Each pregnancy risk category (**A**, **B**, **C**, **D**, or **X**) is explained on the last page of this section.

Remember: All pregnancies have a background risk of 3% or more for a serious birth defect, even when mom doesn't take a drug of any kind. If you are pregnant or planning a pregnancy, always let your healthcare provider know before taking any drug, prescription or non-prescription, or herbal remedy.

The FDA's Pregnancy Risk Categories: A, B, C, D, X

Adapted to the Active Ingredients in Nonprescription drugs

Category A: Controlled studies using the active ingredient in pregnant women have not shown harmful fetal effects throughout pregnancy, and the possibility of fetal harm seems remote. My comment: *Though apparently safe, these active ingredients should still only be used in pregnancy when clearly indicated.*

Category B: Either studies have shown no evidence of fetal harm when using the active ingredient in pregnant animals, but no controlled studies have been done in pregnant women, **or** studies have shown evidence of fetal harm when using the active ingredient in pregnant animals, but controlled studies in pregnant women have not shown evidence of fetal harm. My comment: *These active ingredients should only be used in pregnancy when clearly indicated.*

Category C: Either studies have shown evidence of fetal harm when using the active ingredient in pregnant animals, but no controlled studies have been done in pregnant women, **or** studies using the active ingredient in pregnant animals have not been done, and studies of pregnant women are insufficient to reach a conclusion. These active ingredients should only be used by a pregnant woman if the potential benefit justifies the potential risk of fetal harm, which, in many cases, is unknown. My comment: *It's impossible to calculate the potential risk of fetal harm when, in many cases, it's unknown. Thus, these active ingredients should only be used in pregnancy when clearly needed.*

Category D: Studies have shown evidence of fetal harm when using the active ingredient in pregnant women. However, the potential benefit of using the active ingredient in some life-threatening situations for

mom may outweigh the potential risk of fetal harm. For example, when mom requires cancer treatment or when she has a serious disease for which safer active ingredients cannot be used or are less effective. My comment: *These exceptional indications rarely occur when considering a nonprescription drug in pregnancy.*

Category X: My comment: *Because the risk of fetal harm is too high, no Category X active ingredients have been approved for use in nonprescription drugs.*

Active Ingredients Assigned Two Pregnancy Risk Categories: Some active ingredients have two pregnancy risk categories, depending on which trimester of pregnancy the active ingredient is used. For example, naproxen sodium, the active ingredient in Aleve, belongs to Category **B** when used in the first and second trimesters of pregnancy. If used in the third trimester, however, the active ingredient belongs to Category **D**. My comment: *This means naproxen sodium should not be used in the third trimester unless prescribed by a physician who has advised her patient of the risks involved.*

Section 10: Pain Relief & Fever Reduction

Advil® Migraine Capsules

Active Ingredient:	Pregnancy Risk Category:
Ibuprofen	Ibuprofen has two pregnancy risk categories: **B** when used in the first or second trimesters of pregnancy; **D** if used in the third trimester. (See Helpful Hints below.)

Helpful Hints and Reminders: Each pregnancy risk category (**A**, **B**, **C**, **D**, or **X**) is explained on the last page of this section.

1. Ibuprofen is a member of the non-steroidal, anti-inflammatory family of drugs, or NSAIDs. Members of this family of drugs should not be used during the third trimester of pregnancy (last 12 weeks) unless specifically prescribed by a clinician. See the Appendix for "Non-Steroidal, Anti-Inflammatory Drugs (NSAIDs) in Pregnancy," which describes the serious problems these drugs may cause for unborn babies when taken in the third trimester of pregnancy.

2. Women attempting to conceive should not use any NSAID, including ibuprofen, because of the findings in animals that these drugs may block implantation of the early embryo in the wall of the uterus, in effect preventing pregnancy.

Remember: All pregnancies have a background risk of 3% or more for a serious birth defect, even when mom doesn't take a drug of any kind. If you are pregnant or planning a pregnancy, always let your healthcare provider know before taking any drug, prescription or non-prescription, or herbal remedy.

Advil® PM Caplets & Liqui-Gels®

Active Ingredient:	Pregnancy Risk Category:
Diphenhydramine	B
Ibuprofen	Ibuprofen has two pregnancy risk categories: **B** when used in the first or second trimesters of pregnancy; **D** if used in the third trimester. (See Helpful Hints below.)

Helpful Hints and Reminders: Each pregnancy risk category (**A**, **B**, **C**, **D**, or **X**) is explained on the last page of this section.

1. Ibuprofen is a member of the non-steroidal, anti-inflammatory family of drugs, or NSAIDs. Members of this family of drugs should not be used during the third trimester of pregnancy (last 12 weeks) unless specifically prescribed by a clinician. See the Appendix for "Non-Steroidal, Anti-Inflammatory Drugs (NSAIDs) in Pregnancy," which describes the serious problems these drugs may cause for unborn babies when taken in the third trimester of pregnancy.

2. Women attempting to conceive should not use any NSAID, including ibuprofen, because of the findings in animals that these drugs may block implantation of the early embryo in the wall of the uterus, in effect preventing pregnancy.

Remember: All pregnancies have a background risk of 3% or more for a serious birth defect, even when mom doesn't take a drug of any kind. If you are pregnant or planning a pregnancy, always let your healthcare provider know before taking any drug, prescription or non-prescription, or herbal remedy.

Advil® Tablets, Caplets, Gel Caplets & Liqui-Gel® Caplets

Active Ingredient:	Pregnancy Risk Category:
Ibuprofen	Ibuprofen has two pregnancy risk categories: **B** when used in the first or second trimesters of pregnancy; **D** if used in the third trimester. (See Helpful Hints below.)

Helpful Hints and Reminders: Each pregnancy risk category (**A**, **B**, **C**, **D**, or **X**) is explained on the last page of this section.

1. Ibuprofen is a member of the non-steroidal, anti-inflammatory family of drugs, or NSAIDs. Members of this family of drugs should not be used during the third trimester of pregnancy (last 12 weeks) unless specifically prescribed by a clinician. See the Appendix for "Non-Steroidal, Anti-Inflammatory Drugs (NSAIDs) in Pregnancy," which describes the serious problems these drugs may cause for unborn babies when taken in the third trimester of pregnancy.

2. Women attempting to conceive should not use any NSAID, including ibuprofen, because of the findings in animals that these drugs may block implantation of the early embryo in the wall of the uterus, in effect preventing pregnancy.

Remember: All pregnancies have a background risk of 3% or more for a serious birth defect, even when mom doesn't take a drug of any kind. If you are pregnant or planning a pregnancy, always let your healthcare provider know before taking any drug, prescription or non-prescription, or herbal remedy.

Aleve® All Day Strong Pain Reliever, Fever Reducer, Caplets

Active Ingredient:	Pregnancy Risk Category:
Naproxen sodium	Naproxen sodium has two pregnancy risk categories: **C** when used in the first or second trimesters of pregnancy; **D** if used in the third trimester. (See Helpful Hints below.)

Helpful Hints and Reminders: Each pregnancy risk category (**A**, **B**, **C**, **D**, or **X**) is explained on the last page of this section.

1. Naproxen sodium is a member of the non-steroidal, anti-inflammatory family of drugs, or NSAIDs. Members of this family of drugs should not be used during the third trimester of pregnancy (last 12 weeks) unless specifically prescribed by a clinician. See the Appendix for "Non-Steroidal, Anti-Inflammatory Drugs (NSAIDs) in Pregnancy," which describes the serious problems these drugs may cause for unborn babies when taken in the third trimester of pregnancy.

2. Women attempting to conceive should not use any NSAID, including naproxen sodium, because of the findings in animals that these drugs may block implantation of the early embryo in the wall of the uterus, in effect preventing pregnancy.

Remember: All pregnancies have a background risk of 3% or more for a serious birth defect, even when mom doesn't take a drug of any kind. If you are pregnant or planning a pregnancy, always let your healthcare provider know before taking any drug, prescription or non-prescription, or herbal remedy.

Anacin® Extra Strength Aspirin Free

Active Ingredient:	Pregnancy Risk Category:
Acetaminophen	B

Helpful Hints and Reminders: Each pregnancy risk category (**A**, **B**, **C**, **D**, or **X**) is explained on the last page of this section.

Remember: All pregnancies have a background risk of 3% or more for a serious birth defect, even when mom doesn't take a drug of any kind. If you are pregnant or planning a pregnancy, always let your healthcare provider know before taking any drug, prescription or non-prescription, or herbal remedy.

Anacin® Max Strength Tablets

Active Ingredient:	Pregnancy Risk Category:
Caffeine	B
Aspirin	Aspirin has two pregnancy risk categories: **C** when used in the first or second trimesters of pregnancy; **D** if used in the third trimester. (See Helpful Hints below.)

Helpful Hints and Reminders: Each pregnancy risk category (**A**, **B**, **C**, **D**, or **X**) is explained on the last page of this section.

1. Aspirin is a member of the non-steroidal, anti-inflammatory family of drugs, or NSAIDs. Members of this family of drugs should not be used during the third trimester of pregnancy (last 12 weeks) unless specifically prescribed by a clinician. See the Appendix for "Non-Steroidal, Anti-Inflammatory Drugs (NSAIDs) in Pregnancy," which describes the serious problems these drugs may cause for unborn babies when taken in the third trimester of pregnancy.

2. Women attempting to conceive should not use any NSAID, including aspirin, because of the findings in animals that these drugs may block implantation of the early embryo in the wall of the uterus, in effect preventing pregnancy.

Remember: All pregnancies have a background risk of 3% or more for a serious birth defect, even when mom doesn't take a drug of any kind. If you are pregnant or planning a pregnancy, always let your healthcare provider know before taking any drug, prescription or non-prescription, or herbal remedy.

Anacin® Regular Strength Tablets & Caplets

Active Ingredient:	Pregnancy Risk Category:
Caffeine	B
Aspirin	Aspirin has two pregnancy risk categories: **C** when used in the first or second trimesters of pregnancy; **D** if used in the third trimester. (See Helpful Hints below.)

Helpful Hints and Reminders: Each pregnancy risk category (**A**, **B**, **C**, **D**, or **X**) is explained on the last page of this section.

1. Aspirin is a member of the non-steroidal, anti-inflammatory family of drugs, or NSAIDs. Members of this family of drugs should not be used during the third trimester of pregnancy (last 12 weeks) unless specifically prescribed by a clinician. See the Appendix for "Non-Steroidal, Anti-Inflammatory Drugs (NSAIDs) in Pregnancy," which describes the serious problems these drugs may cause for unborn babies when taken in the third trimester of pregnancy.

2. Women attempting to conceive should not use any NSAID, including aspirin, because of the findings in animals that these drugs may block implantation of the early embryo in the wall of the uterus, in effect preventing pregnancy.

Remember: All pregnancies have a background risk of 3% or more for a serious birth defect, even when mom doesn't take a drug of any kind. If you are pregnant or planning a pregnancy, always let your healthcare provider know before taking any drug, prescription or non-prescription, or herbal remedy.

Ascriptin® Maximum Strength Pain Reliever Caplets

Active Ingredient:	Pregnancy Risk Category:
Aluminum hydroxide	C

(continued)

Calcium carbonate	C
Magnesium hydroxide	C
Aspirin	Aspirin has two pregnancy risk categories: **C** when used in the first or second trimesters of pregnancy; **D** if used in the third trimester. (See Helpful Hints below.)

Helpful Hints and Reminders: Each pregnancy risk category (**A**, **B**, **C**, **D**, or **X**) is explained on the last page of this section.

1. Aspirin is a member of the non-steroidal, anti-inflammatory family of drugs, or NSAIDs. Members of this family of drugs should not be used during the third trimester of pregnancy (last 12 weeks) unless specifically prescribed by a clinician. See the Appendix for "Non-Steroidal, Anti-Inflammatory Drugs (NSAIDs) in Pregnancy," which describes the serious problems these drugs may cause for unborn babies when taken in the third trimester of pregnancy.

2. Women attempting to conceive should not use any NSAID, including aspirin, because of the findings in animals that these drugs may block implantation of the early embryo in the wall of the uterus, in effect preventing pregnancy.

Remember: All pregnancies have a background risk of 3% or more for a serious birth defect, even when mom doesn't take a drug of any kind. If you are pregnant or planning a pregnancy, always let your healthcare provider know before taking any drug, prescription or non-prescription, or herbal remedy.

Ascriptin® Tablets Regular Strength

Active Ingredient:	Pregnancy Risk Category:
Aluminum hydroxide	C
Calcium carbonate	C
Magnesium hydroxide	C

(continued)

| Aspirin | Aspirin has two pregnancy risk categories: **C** when used in the first or second trimesters of pregnancy; **D** if used in the third trimester. (See Helpful Hints below.) |

Helpful Hints and Reminders: Each pregnancy risk category (**A**, **B**, **C**, **D**, or **X**) is explained on the last page of this section.

1. Aspirin is a member of the non-steroidal, anti-inflammatory family of drugs, or NSAIDs. Members of this family of drugs should not be used during the third trimester of pregnancy (last 12 weeks) unless specifically prescribed by a clinician. See the Appendix for "Non-Steroidal, Anti-Inflammatory Drugs (NSAIDs) in Pregnancy," which describes the serious problems these drugs may cause for unborn babies when taken in the third trimester of pregnancy.

2. Women attempting to conceive should not use any NSAID, including aspirin, because of the findings in animals that these drugs may block implantation of the early embryo in the wall of the uterus, in effect preventing pregnancy.

Remember: All pregnancies have a background risk of 3% or more for a serious birth defect, even when mom doesn't take a drug of any kind. If you are pregnant or planning a pregnancy, always let your healthcare provider know before taking any drug, prescription or non-prescription, or herbal remedy.

Bayer® AM Extra Strength Aspirin & Alertness Aid Tablets

Active Ingredient:	Pregnancy Risk Category:
Caffeine	**B**
Aspirin	Aspirin has two pregnancy risk categories: **C** when used in the first or second trimesters of pregnancy; **D** if used in the third trimester. (See Helpful Hints on the next page.)

Bayer® Aspirin Extra Strength

Helpful Hints and Reminders: Each pregnancy risk category (**A**, **B**, **C**, **D**, or **X**) is explained on the last page of this section.

1. Aspirin is a member of the non-steroidal, anti-inflammatory family of drugs, or NSAIDs. Members of this family of drugs should not be used during the third trimester of pregnancy (last 12 weeks) unless specifically prescribed by a clinician. See the Appendix for "Non-Steroidal, Anti-Inflammatory Drugs (NSAIDs) in Pregnancy," which describes the serious problems these drugs may cause for unborn babies when taken in the third trimester of pregnancy.

2. Women attempting to conceive should not use any NSAID, including aspirin, because of the findings in animals that these drugs may block implantation of the early embryo in the wall of the uterus, in effect preventing pregnancy.

Remember: All pregnancies have a background risk of 3% or more for a serious birth defect, even when mom doesn't take a drug of any kind. If you are pregnant or planning a pregnancy, always let your healthcare provider know before taking any drug, prescription or non-prescription, or herbal remedy.

Bayer® Aspirin Extra Strength

Active Ingredient:	Pregnancy Risk Category:
Aspirin	Aspirin has two pregnancy risk categories: **C** when used in the first or second trimesters of pregnancy; **D** if used in the third trimester. (See Helpful Hints below.)

Helpful Hints and Reminders: Each pregnancy risk category (**A**, **B**, **C**, **D**, or **X**) is explained on the last page of this section.

1. Aspirin is a member of the non-steroidal, anti-inflammatory family of drugs, or NSAIDs. Members of this family of drugs should not be used during the third trimester of pregnancy (last 12 weeks) unless specifically prescribed by a clinician. See the Appendix for "Non-Steroidal, Anti-Inflammatory Drugs

(NSAIDs) in Pregnancy," which describes the serious problems these drugs may cause for unborn babies when taken in the third trimester of pregnancy.

2. Women attempting to conceive should not use any NSAID, including aspirin, because of the findings in animals that these drugs may block implantation of the early embryo in the wall of the uterus, in effect preventing pregnancy.

Remember: All pregnancies have a background risk of 3% or more for a serious birth defect, even when mom doesn't take a drug of any kind. If you are pregnant or planning a pregnancy, always let your healthcare provider know before taking any drug, prescription or non-prescription, or herbal remedy.

Bayer® Aspirin Tablets

Active Ingredient:	Pregnancy Risk Category:
Aspirin	Aspirin has two pregnancy risk categories: **C** when used in the first or second trimesters of pregnancy; **D** if used in the third trimester. (See Helpful Hints below.)

Helpful Hints and Reminders: Each pregnancy risk category (**A**, **B**, **C**, **D**, or **X**) is explained on the last page of this section.

1. Aspirin is a member of the non-steroidal, anti-inflammatory family of drugs, or NSAIDs. Members of this family of drugs should not be used during the third trimester of pregnancy (last 12 weeks) unless specifically prescribed by a clinician. See the Appendix for "Non-Steroidal, Anti-Inflammatory Drugs (NSAIDs) in Pregnancy," which describes the serious problems these drugs may cause for unborn babies when taken in the third trimester of pregnancy.

2. Women attempting to conceive should not use any NSAID, including aspirin, because of the findings in animals that these drugs may block implantation of the early embryo in the wall of the uterus, in effect preventing pregnancy.

Remember: All pregnancies have a background risk of 3% or more for a serious birth defect, even when mom doesn't take a drug of any kind. If you are pregnant or planning a pregnancy, always let your healthcare provider know before taking any drug, prescription or non-prescription, or herbal remedy.

Bayer® Chewable Aspirin, Orange and Cherry

Active Ingredient:	Pregnancy Risk Category:
Aspirin	Aspirin has two pregnancy risk categories: **C** when used in the first or second trimesters of pregnancy; **D** if used in the third trimester. (See Helpful Hints below.)

Helpful Hints and Reminders: Each pregnancy risk category (**A**, **B**, **C**, **D**, or **X**) is explained on the last page of this section.

1. Aspirin is a member of the non-steroidal, anti-inflammatory family of drugs, or NSAIDs. Members of this family of drugs should not be used during the third trimester of pregnancy (last 12 weeks) unless specifically prescribed by a clinician. See the Appendix for "Non-Steroidal, Anti-Inflammatory Drugs (NSAIDs) in Pregnancy," which describes the serious problems these drugs may cause for unborn babies when taken in the third trimester of pregnancy.

2. Women attempting to conceive should not use any NSAID, including aspirin, because of the findings in animals that these drugs may block implantation of the early embryo in the wall of the uterus, in effect preventing pregnancy.

Remember: All pregnancies have a background risk of 3% or more for a serious birth defect, even when mom doesn't take a drug of any kind. If you are pregnant or planning a pregnancy, always let your healthcare provider know before taking any drug, prescription or non-prescription, or herbal remedy.

Bayer® Extra Strength Back & Body Pain

Active Ingredient:	Pregnancy Risk Category:
Caffeine	B
Aspirin	Aspirin has two pregnancy risk categories: **C** when used in the first or second trimesters of pregnancy; **D** if used in the third trimester. (See Helpful Hints below.)

Helpful Hints and Reminders: Each pregnancy risk category (**A**, **B**, **C**, **D**, or **X**) is explained on the last page of this section.

1. Aspirin is a member of the non-steroidal, anti-inflammatory family of drugs, or NSAIDs. Members of this family of drugs should not be used during the third trimester of pregnancy (last 12 weeks) unless specifically prescribed by a clinician. See the Appendix for "Non-Steroidal, Anti-Inflammatory Drugs (NSAIDs) in Pregnancy," which describes the serious problems these drugs may cause for unborn babies when taken in the third trimester of pregnancy.

2. Women attempting to conceive should not use any NSAID, including aspirin, because of the findings in animals that these drugs may block implantation of the early embryo in the wall of the uterus, in effect preventing pregnancy.

Remember: All pregnancies have a background risk of 3% or more for a serious birth defect, even when mom doesn't take a drug of any kind. If you are pregnant or planning a pregnancy, always let your healthcare provider know before taking any drug, prescription or non-prescription, or herbal remedy.

Bayer® Extra Strength Plus

Active Ingredient:	Pregnancy Risk Category:
Calcium carbonate	C

(continued)

| Aspirin | Aspirin has two pregnancy risk categories: **C** when used in the first or second trimesters of pregnancy; **D** if used in the third trimester. (See Helpful Hints below.) |

Helpful Hints and Reminders: Each pregnancy risk category (**A**, **B**, **C**, **D**, or **X**) is explained on the last page of this section.

1. Aspirin is a member of the non-steroidal, anti-inflammatory family of drugs, or NSAIDs. Members of this family of drugs should not be used during the third trimester of pregnancy (last 12 weeks) unless specifically prescribed by a clinician. See the Appendix for "Non-Steroidal, Anti-Inflammatory Drugs (NSAIDs) in Pregnancy," which describes the serious problems these drugs may cause for unborn babies when taken in the third trimester of pregnancy.

2. Women attempting to conceive should not use any NSAID, including aspirin, because of the findings in animals that these drugs may block implantation of the early embryo in the wall of the uterus, in effect preventing pregnancy.

Remember: All pregnancies have a background risk of 3% or more for a serious birth defect, even when mom doesn't take a drug of any kind. If you are pregnant or planning a pregnancy, always let your healthcare provider know before taking any drug, prescription or non-prescription, or herbal remedy.

Bayer® PM

Active Ingredient:	Pregnancy Risk Category:
Diphenhydramine citrate	**B**
Aspirin	Aspirin has two pregnancy risk categories: **C** when used in the first or second trimesters of pregnancy; **D** if used in the third trimester. (See Helpful Hints on the next page.)

Helpful Hints and Reminders: Each pregnancy risk category (**A**, **B**, **C**, **D**, or **X**) is explained on the last page of this section.

1. Aspirin is a member of the non-steroidal, anti-inflammatory family of drugs, or NSAIDs. Members of this family of drugs should not be used during the third trimester of pregnancy (last 12 weeks) unless specifically prescribed by a clinician. See the Appendix for "Non-Steroidal, Anti-Inflammatory Drugs (NSAIDs) in Pregnancy," which describes the serious problems these drugs may cause for unborn babies when taken in the third trimester of pregnancy.

2. Women attempting to conceive should not use any NSAID, including aspirin, because of the findings in animals that these drugs may block implantation of the early embryo in the wall of the uterus, in effect preventing pregnancy.

Remember: All pregnancies have a background risk of 3% or more for a serious birth defect, even when mom doesn't take a drug of any kind. If you are pregnant or planning a pregnancy, always let your healthcare provider know before taking any drug, prescription or non-prescription, or herbal remedy.

Bayer® Quick Release Crystals

Active Ingredient:	Pregnancy Risk Category:
Caffeine	**B**
Aspirin	Aspirin has two pregnancy risk categories: **C** when used in the first or second trimesters of pregnancy; **D** if used in the third trimester. (See Helpful Hints below.)

Helpful Hints and Reminders: Each pregnancy risk category (**A**, **B**, **C**, **D**, or **X**) is explained on the last page of this section.

1. Aspirin is a member of the non-steroidal, anti-inflammatory family of drugs, or NSAIDs. Members of this family of drugs should not be used during the third trimester of pregnancy (last

12 weeks) unless specifically prescribed by a clinician. See the Appendix for "Non-Steroidal, Anti-Inflammatory Drugs (NSAIDs) in Pregnancy," which describes the serious problems these drugs may cause for unborn babies when taken in the third trimester of pregnancy.

2. Women attempting to conceive should not use any NSAID, including aspirin, because of the findings in animals that these drugs may block implantation of the early embryo in the wall of the uterus, in effect preventing pregnancy.

Remember: All pregnancies have a background risk of 3% or more for a serious birth defect, even when mom doesn't take a drug of any kind. If you are pregnant or planning a pregnancy, always let your healthcare provider know before taking any drug, prescription or non-prescription, or herbal remedy.

Bayer® Women's Low Dose Aspirin

Active Ingredient:	Pregnancy Risk Category:
Calcium carbonate	C
Aspirin	Aspirin has two pregnancy risk categories: **C** when used in the first or second trimesters of pregnancy; **D** if used in the third trimester. (See Helpful Hints below.)

Helpful Hints and Reminders: Each pregnancy risk category (**A**, **B**, **C**, **D**, or **X**) is explained on the last page of this section.

1. Aspirin is a member of the non-steroidal, anti-inflammatory family of drugs, or NSAIDs. Members of this family of drugs should not be used during the third trimester of pregnancy (last 12 weeks) unless specifically prescribed by a clinician. See the Appendix for "Non-Steroidal, Anti-Inflammatory Drugs (NSAIDs) in Pregnancy," which describes the serious problems these drugs may cause for unborn babies when taken in the third trimester of pregnancy.

2. Women attempting to conceive should not use any NSAID, including aspirin, because of the findings in animals that these drugs may block implantation of the early embryo in the wall of the uterus, in effect preventing pregnancy.

Remember: All pregnancies have a background risk of 3% or more for a serious birth defect, even when mom doesn't take a drug of any kind. If you are pregnant or planning a pregnancy, always let your healthcare provider know before taking any drug, prescription or non-prescription, or herbal remedy.

Bufferin® Regular and Extra Strength Tablets

Active Ingredient:	Pregnancy Risk Category:
Aspirin	Aspirin has two pregnancy risk categories: **C** when used in the first or second trimesters of pregnancy; **D** if used in the third trimester. (See Helpful Hints below.)

Helpful Hints and Reminders: Each pregnancy risk category (**A**, **B**, **C**, **D**, or **X**) is explained on the last page of this section.

1. Aspirin is a member of the non-steroidal, anti-inflammatory family of drugs, or NSAIDs. Members of this family of drugs should not be used during the third trimester of pregnancy (last 12 weeks) unless specifically prescribed by a clinician. See the Appendix for "Non-Steroidal, Anti-Inflammatory Drugs (NSAIDs) in Pregnancy," which describes the serious problems these drugs may cause for unborn babies when taken in the third trimester of pregnancy.

2. Women attempting to conceive should not use any NSAID, including aspirin, because of the findings in animals that these drugs may block implantation of the early embryo in the wall of the uterus, in effect preventing pregnancy.

Remember: All pregnancies have a background risk of 3% or more for a serious birth defect, even when mom doesn't take a drug of any kind. If you are pregnant or planning a pregnancy, always let your healthcare

provider know before taking any drug, prescription or non-prescription, or herbal remedy.

CVS® Arthritis Pain Relief Caplets Easy Open Bottle

Active Ingredient:	Pregnancy Risk Category:
Acetaminophen	B

Helpful Hints and Reminders: Each pregnancy risk category (**A**, **B**, **C**, **D**, or **X**) is explained on the last page of this section.

Remember: All pregnancies have a background risk of 3% or more for a serious birth defect, even when mom doesn't take a drug of any kind. If you are pregnant or planning a pregnancy, always let your healthcare provider know before taking any drug, prescription or non-prescription, or herbal remedy.

CVS® Aspirin 325 Mg Coated Tablets Regular Strength

Active Ingredient:	Pregnancy Risk Category:
Aspirin	Aspirin has two pregnancy risk categories: **C** when used in the first or second trimesters of pregnancy; **D** if used in the third trimester. (See Helpful Hints below.)

Helpful Hints and Reminders: Each pregnancy risk category (**A**, **B**, **C**, **D**, or **X**) is explained on the last page of this section.

1. Aspirin is a member of the non-steroidal, anti-inflammatory family of drugs, or NSAIDs. Members of this family of drugs should not be used during the third trimester of pregnancy (last 12 weeks) unless specifically prescribed by a clinician. See the Appendix for "Non-Steroidal, Anti-Inflammatory Drugs (NSAIDs) in Pregnancy," which describes the serious problems these drugs may cause for unborn babies when taken in the third trimester of pregnancy.

2. Women attempting to conceive should not use any NSAID, including aspirin, because of the findings in animals that these drugs may block implantation of the early embryo in the wall of the uterus, in effect preventing pregnancy.

Remember: All pregnancies have a background risk of 3% or more for a serious birth defect, even when mom doesn't take a drug of any kind. If you are pregnant or planning a pregnancy, always let your healthcare provider know before taking any drug, prescription or non-prescription, or herbal remedy.

CVS® Aspirin Free Pain Relief PM

Active Ingredient:	Pregnancy Risk Category:
Acetaminophen	B
Diphenhydramine citrate	B

Helpful Hints and Reminders: Each pregnancy risk category (**A**, **B**, **C**, **D**, or **X**) is explained on the last page of this section.

Remember: All pregnancies have a background risk of 3% or more for a serious birth defect, even when mom doesn't take a drug of any kind. If you are pregnant or planning a pregnancy, always let your healthcare provider know before taking any drug, prescription or non-prescription, or herbal remedy.

CVS® Extra Strength Non-Aspirin PM Caplets

Active Ingredient:	Pregnancy Risk Category:
Acetaminophen	B
Diphenhydramine Hcl	B

Helpful Hints and Reminders: Each pregnancy risk category (**A**, **B**, **C**, **D**, or **X**) is explained on the last page of this section.

Remember: All pregnancies have a background risk of 3% or more for a serious birth defect, even when mom doesn't take a drug of any kind. If you are pregnant or planning a pregnancy, always let your healthcare provider know before taking any drug, prescription or non-prescription, or herbal remedy.

CVS® Extra Strength Pain Relief PM Geltabs

Active Ingredient:	Pregnancy Risk Category:
Acetaminophen	B
Diphenhydramine Hcl	B

Helpful Hints and Reminders: Each pregnancy risk category (**A**, **B**, **C**, **D**, or **X**) is explained on the last page of this section.

Remember: All pregnancies have a background risk of 3% or more for a serious birth defect, even when mom doesn't take a drug of any kind. If you are pregnant or planning a pregnancy, always let your healthcare provider know before taking any drug, prescription or non-prescription, or herbal remedy.

CVS® Extra Strength Pain Relief PM Rapid Release Gelcaps

Active Ingredient:	Pregnancy Risk Category:
Acetaminophen	B
Diphenhydramine Hcl	B

Helpful Hints and Reminders: Each pregnancy risk category (**A**, **B**, **C**, **D**, or **X**) is explained on the last page of this section.

Remember: All pregnancies have a background risk of 3% or more for a serious birth defect, even when mom doesn't take a drug of any kind. If you are pregnant or planning a pregnancy, always let your healthcare provider know before taking any drug, prescription or non-prescription, or herbal remedy.

CVS® Headache Relief Coated Tablets Added Strength

Active Ingredient:	Pregnancy Risk Category:
Acetaminophen	B
Caffeine	B

(*continued*)

Aspirin	Aspirin has two pregnancy risk categories: **C** when used in the first or second trimesters of pregnancy; **D** if used in the third trimester. (See Helpful Hints below.)

Helpful Hints and Reminders: Each pregnancy risk category (**A**, **B**, **C**, **D**, or **X**) is explained on the last page of this section.

1. Aspirin is a member of the non-steroidal, anti-inflammatory family of drugs, or NSAIDs. Members of this family of drugs should not be used during the third trimester of pregnancy (last 12 weeks) unless specifically prescribed by a clinician. See the Appendix for "Non-Steroidal, Anti-Inflammatory Drugs (NSAIDs) in Pregnancy," which describes the serious problems these drugs may cause for unborn babies when taken in the third trimester of pregnancy.

2. Women attempting to conceive should not use any NSAID, including aspirin, because of the findings in animals that these drugs may block implantation of the early embryo in the wall of the uterus, in effect preventing pregnancy.

Remember: All pregnancies have a background risk of 3% or more for a serious birth defect, even when mom doesn't take a drug of any kind. If you are pregnant or planning a pregnancy, always let your healthcare provider know before taking any drug, prescription or non-prescription, or herbal remedy.

CVS® Ibuprofen PM Pain Reliever Coated Caplets 200 Mg

Active Ingredient:	Pregnancy Risk Category:
Diphenhydramine citrate	**B**
Ibuprofen	Ibuprofen has two pregnancy risk categories: **B** when used in the first or second trimesters of pregnancy; **D** if used in the third trimester. (See Helpful Hints on the next page.)

Helpful Hints and Reminders: Each pregnancy risk category (**A**, **B**, **C**, **D**, or **X**) is explained on the last page of this section.

1. Ibuprofen is a member of the non-steroidal, anti-inflammatory family of drugs, or NSAIDs. Members of this family of drugs should not be used during the third trimester of pregnancy (last 12 weeks) unless specifically prescribed by a clinician. See the Appendix for "Non-Steroidal, Anti-Inflammatory Drugs (NSAIDs) in Pregnancy," which describes the serious problems these drugs may cause for unborn babies when taken in the third trimester of pregnancy.

2. Women attempting to conceive should not use any NSAID, including ibuprofen, because of the findings in animals that these drugs may block implantation of the early embryo in the wall of the uterus, in effect preventing pregnancy.

Remember: All pregnancies have a background risk of 3% or more for a serious birth defect, even when mom doesn't take a drug of any kind. If you are pregnant or planning a pregnancy, always let your healthcare provider know before taking any drug, prescription or non-prescription, or herbal remedy.

CVS® Migraine Relief Caplets

Active Ingredient:	Pregnancy Risk Category:
Acetaminophen	B
Caffeine	C
Aspirin	Aspirin has two pregnancy risk categories: **C** when used in the first or second trimesters of pregnancy; **D** if used in the third trimester. (See Helpful Hints below.)

Helpful Hints and Reminders: Each pregnancy risk category (**A**, **B**, **C**, **D**, or **X**) is explained on the last page of this section.

1. Aspirin is a member of the non-steroidal, anti-inflammatory family of drugs, or NSAIDs. Members of this family of drugs should not be used during the third trimester of pregnancy (last

12 weeks) unless specifically prescribed by a clinician. See the Appendix for "Non-Steroidal, Anti-Inflammatory Drugs (NSAIDs) in Pregnancy," which describes the serious problems these drugs may cause for unborn babies when taken in the third trimester of pregnancy.

2. Women attempting to conceive should not use any NSAID, including aspirin, because of the findings in animals that these drugs may block implantation of the early embryo in the wall of the uterus, in effect preventing pregnancy.

Remember: All pregnancies have a background risk of 3% or more for a serious birth defect, even when mom doesn't take a drug of any kind. If you are pregnant or planning a pregnancy, always let your healthcare provider know before taking any drug, prescription or non-prescription, or herbal remedy.

CVS® Pain Relief PM & Pain Relief Caplets Extra Strength

Active Ingredient:	Pregnancy Risk Category:
Pain Reliever PM:	
Acetaminophen	B
Diphenhydramine Hcl	B
Pain Reliever:	
Acetaminophen	B

Helpful Hints and Reminders: Each pregnancy risk category (**A**, **B**, **C**, **D**, or **X**) is explained on the last page of this section.

Remember: All pregnancies have a background risk of 3% or more for a serious birth defect, even when mom doesn't take a drug of any kind. If you are pregnant or planning a pregnancy, always let your healthcare provider know before taking any drug, prescription or non-prescription, or herbal remedy.

Equate® Acetaminophen Extra Strength 500 Mg/Non-Aspirin/Easy Tabs Pain Reliever

Active Ingredient:	Pregnancy Risk Category:
Acetaminophen	B

Helpful Hints and Reminders: Each pregnancy risk category (**A**, **B**, **C**, **D**, or **X**) is explained on the last page of this section.

Remember: All pregnancies have a background risk of 3% or more for a serious birth defect, even when mom doesn't take a drug of any kind. If you are pregnant or planning a pregnancy, always let your healthcare provider know before taking any drug, prescription or non-prescription, or herbal remedy.

Equate® Allergy/Sinus Headache Pain Reliever Caplets

Active Ingredient:	Pregnancy Risk Category:
Diphenhydramine Hcl	B
Acetaminophen	B
Phenylephrine Hcl	C

Helpful Hints and Reminders: Each pregnancy risk category (**A**, **B**, **C**, **D**, or **X**) is explained on the last page of this section.

Remember: All pregnancies have a background risk of 3% or more for a serious birth defect, even when mom doesn't take a drug of any kind. If you are pregnant or planning a pregnancy, always let your healthcare provider know before taking any drug, prescription or non-prescription, or herbal remedy.

Equate® Arthritis Pain Reliever Caplets

Active Ingredient:	Pregnancy Risk Category:
Acetaminophen	B

Helpful Hints and Reminders: Each pregnancy risk category (**A**, **B**, **C**, **D**, or **X**) is explained on the last page of this section.

Remember: All pregnancies have a background risk of 3% or more for a serious birth defect, even when mom doesn't take a drug of any kind. If you are pregnant or planning a pregnancy, always let your healthcare provider know before taking any drug, prescription or non-prescription, or herbal remedy.

Equate® Aspirin Tablets 325 Mg Pain Reliever/Fever Reducer

Active Ingredient:	Pregnancy Risk Category:
Aspirin	Aspirin has two pregnancy risk categories: **C** when used in the first or second trimesters of pregnancy; **D** if used in the third trimester. (See Helpful Hints below.)

Helpful Hints and Reminders: Each pregnancy risk category (**A**, **B**, **C**, **D**, or **X**) is explained on the last page of this section.

1. Aspirin is a member of the non-steroidal, anti-inflammatory family of drugs, or NSAIDs. Members of this family of drugs should not be used during the third trimester of pregnancy (last 12 weeks) unless specifically prescribed by a clinician. See the Appendix for "Non-Steroidal, Anti-Inflammatory Drugs (NSAIDs) in Pregnancy," which describes the serious problems these drugs may cause for unborn babies when taken in the third trimester of pregnancy.

2. Women attempting to conceive should not use any NSAID, including aspirin, because of the findings in animals that these drugs may block implantation of the early embryo in the wall of the uterus, in effect preventing pregnancy.

Remember: All pregnancies have a background risk of 3% or more for a serious birth defect, even when mom doesn't take a drug of any kind. If you are pregnant or planning a pregnancy, always let your healthcare provider know before taking any drug, prescription or non-prescription, or herbal remedy.

Equate® Extra Strength Caplets Pain Reliever/Fever Reducer

Active Ingredient:	Pregnancy Risk Category:
Acetaminophen	B

Helpful Hints and Reminders: Each pregnancy risk category (**A**, **B**, **C**, **D**, or **X**) is explained on the last page of this section.

Remember: All pregnancies have a background risk of 3% or more for a serious birth defect, even when mom doesn't take a drug of any kind. If you are pregnant or planning a pregnancy, always let your healthcare provider know before taking any drug, prescription or non-prescription, or herbal remedy.

Equate® Extra Strength Pain Reliever PM Caplets

Active Ingredient:	Pregnancy Risk Category:
Acetaminophen	B
Diphenhydramine Hcl	B

Helpful Hints and Reminders: Each pregnancy risk category (**A**, **B**, **C**, **D**, or **X**) is explained on the last page of this section.

Remember: All pregnancies have a background risk of 3% or more for a serious birth defect, even when mom doesn't take a drug of any kind. If you are pregnant or planning a pregnancy, always let your healthcare provider know before taking any drug, prescription or non-prescription, or herbal remedy.

Equate® Ibuprofen 200 Mg Tablets

Active Ingredient:	Pregnancy Risk Category:
Ibuprofen	Ibuprofen has two pregnancy risk categories: **B** when used in the first or second trimesters of pregnancy; **D** if used in the third trimester. (See Helpful Hints on the next page.)

Helpful Hints and Reminders: Each pregnancy risk category (**A**, **B**, **C**, **D**, or **X**) is explained on the last page of this section.

1. Ibuprofen is a member of the non-steroidal, anti-inflammatory family of drugs, or NSAIDs. Members of this family of drugs should not be used during the third trimester of pregnancy (last 12 weeks) unless specifically prescribed by a clinician. See the Appendix for "Non-Steroidal, Anti-Inflammatory Drugs (NSAIDs) in Pregnancy," which describes the serious problems these drugs may cause for unborn babies when taken in the third trimester of pregnancy.

2. Women attempting to conceive should not use any NSAID, including ibuprofen, because of the findings in animals that these drugs may block implantation of the early embryo in the wall of the uterus, in effect preventing pregnancy.

Remember: All pregnancies have a background risk of 3% or more for a serious birth defect, even when mom doesn't take a drug of any kind. If you are pregnant or planning a pregnancy, always let your healthcare provider know before taking any drug, prescription or non-prescription, or herbal remedy.

Equate® Ibuprofen PM Caplets Pain Reliever/Sleep Aid

Active Ingredient:	Pregnancy Risk Category:
Diphenhydramine citrate	B
Ibuprofen	Ibuprofen has two pregnancy risk categories: **B** when used in the first or second trimesters of pregnancy; **D** if used in the third trimester. (See Helpful Hints below.)

Helpful Hints and Reminders: Each pregnancy risk category (**A**, **B**, **C**, **D**, or **X**) is explained on the last page of this section.

1. Ibuprofen is a member of the non-steroidal, anti-inflammatory family of drugs, or NSAIDs. Members of this family of drugs

Equate® Ibuprofen Softgels 200 Mg Pain Reliever/Fever Reducer **231**

> should not be used during the third trimester of pregnancy (last 12 weeks) unless specifically prescribed by a clinician. See the Appendix for "Non-Steroidal, Anti-Inflammatory Drugs (NSAIDs) in Pregnancy," which describes the serious problems these drugs may cause for unborn babies when taken in the third trimester of pregnancy.
>
> 2. Women attempting to conceive should not use any NSAID, including ibuprofen, because of the findings in animals that these drugs may block implantation of the early embryo in the wall of the uterus, in effect preventing pregnancy.

Remember: All pregnancies have a background risk of 3% or more for a serious birth defect, even when mom doesn't take a drug of any kind. If you are pregnant or planning a pregnancy, always let your healthcare provider know before taking any drug, prescription or non-prescription, or herbal remedy.

Equate® Ibuprofen Softgels 200 Mg Pain Reliever/Fever Reducer

Active Ingredient:	Pregnancy Risk Category:
Ibuprofen	Ibuprofen has two pregnancy risk categories: **B** when used in the first or second trimesters of pregnancy; **D** if used in the third trimester. (See Helpful Hints below.)

Helpful Hints and Reminders: Each pregnancy risk category (**A**, **B**, **C**, **D**, or **X**) is explained on the last page of this section.

> 1. Ibuprofen is a member of the non-steroidal, anti-inflammatory family of drugs, or NSAIDs. Members of this family of drugs should not be used during the third trimester of pregnancy (last 12 weeks) unless specifically prescribed by a clinician. See the Appendix for "Non-Steroidal, Anti-Inflammatory Drugs (NSAIDs) in Pregnancy," which describes the serious problems these drugs may cause for unborn babies when taken in the third trimester of pregnancy.

2. Women attempting to conceive should not use any NSAID, including ibuprofen, because of the findings in animals that these drugs may block implantation of the early embryo in the wall of the uterus, in effect preventing pregnancy.

Remember: All pregnancies have a background risk of 3% or more for a serious birth defect, even when mom doesn't take a drug of any kind. If you are pregnant or planning a pregnancy, always let your healthcare provider know before taking any drug, prescription or non-prescription, or herbal remedy.

Equate® Naproxen Sodium Tablets 220 Mg Pain Reliever/Fever Reducer

Active Ingredient:	Pregnancy Risk Category:
Naproxen sodium	Naproxen sodium has two pregnancy risk categories: **C** when used in the first or second trimesters of pregnancy; **D** if used in the third trimester. (See Helpful Hints below.)

Helpful Hints and Reminders: Each pregnancy risk category (**A**, **B**, **C**, **D**, or **X**) is explained on the last page of this section.

1. Naproxen sodium is a member of the non-steroidal, anti-inflammatory family of drugs, or NSAIDs. Members of this family of drugs should not be used during the third trimester of pregnancy (last 12 weeks) unless specifically prescribed by a clinician. See the Appendix for "Non-Steroidal, Anti-Inflammatory Drugs (NSAIDs) in Pregnancy," which describes the serious problems these drugs may cause for unborn babies when taken in the third trimester of pregnancy.

2. Women attempting to conceive should not use any NSAID, including naproxen sodium, because of the findings in animals that these drugs may block implantation of the early embryo in the wall of the uterus, in effect preventing pregnancy.

Remember: All pregnancies have a background risk of 3% or more for a serious birth defect, even when mom doesn't take a drug of any kind.

If you are pregnant or planning a pregnancy, always let your healthcare provider know before taking any drug, prescription or non-prescription, or herbal remedy.

Equate® Original Effervescent Antacid & Pain Relief

Active Ingredient:	Pregnancy Risk Category:
Sodium bicarbonate	C
Citric acid	**Risk is undetermined.** The FDA has not assigned a pregnancy risk category to this drug.
Aspirin	Aspirin has two pregnancy risk categories: **C** when used in the first or second trimesters of pregnancy; **D** if used in the third trimester. (See Helpful Hints below.)

Helpful Hints and Reminders: Each pregnancy risk category (**A**, **B**, **C**, **D**, or **X**) is explained on the last page of this section.

1. Aspirin is a member of the non-steroidal, anti-inflammatory family of drugs, or NSAIDs. Members of this family of drugs should not be used during the third trimester of pregnancy (last 12 weeks) unless specifically prescribed by a clinician. See the Appendix for "Non-Steroidal, Anti-Inflammatory Drugs (NSAIDs) in Pregnancy," which describes the serious problems these drugs may cause for unborn babies when taken in the third trimester of pregnancy.

2. Women attempting to conceive should not use any NSAID, including aspirin, because of the findings in animals that these drugs may block implantation of the early embryo in the wall of the uterus, in effect preventing pregnancy.

Remember: All pregnancies have a background risk of 3% or more for a serious birth defect, even when mom doesn't take a drug of any kind. If you are pregnant or planning a pregnancy, always let your healthcare provider know before taking any drug, prescription or non-prescription, or herbal remedy.

Excedrin® Back and Body Caplets

Active Ingredient:	Pregnancy Risk Category:
Acetaminophen	B
Aspirin	Aspirin has two pregnancy risk categories: **C** when used in the first or second trimesters of pregnancy; **D** if used in the third trimester. (See Helpful Hints below.)

Helpful Hints and Reminders: Each pregnancy risk category (**A**, **B**, **C**, **D**, or **X**) is explained on the last page of this section.

1. Aspirin is a member of the non-steroidal, anti-inflammatory family of drugs, or NSAIDs. Members of this family of drugs should not be used during the third trimester of pregnancy (last 12 weeks) unless specifically prescribed by a clinician. See the Appendix for "Non-Steroidal, Anti-Inflammatory Drugs (NSAIDs) in Pregnancy," which describes the serious problems these drugs may cause for unborn babies when taken in the third trimester of pregnancy.

2. Women attempting to conceive should not use any NSAID, including aspirin, because of the findings in animals that these drugs may block implantation of the early embryo in the wall of the uterus, in effect preventing pregnancy.

Remember: All pregnancies have a background risk of 3% or more for a serious birth defect, even when mom doesn't take a drug of any kind. If you are pregnant or planning a pregnancy, always let your healthcare provider know before taking any drug, prescription or non-prescription, or herbal remedy.

Excedrin® Extra Strength Caplets, Tablets, and Geltabs

Active Ingredient:	Pregnancy Risk Category:
Acetaminophen	B

(continued)

Caffeine	B
Aspirin	Aspirin has two pregnancy risk categories: **C** when used in the first or second trimesters of pregnancy; **D** if used in the third trimester. (See Helpful Hints below.)

Helpful Hints and Reminders: Each pregnancy risk category (**A**, **B**, **C**, **D**, or **X**) is explained on the last page of this section.

1. Aspirin is a member of the non-steroidal, anti-inflammatory family of drugs, or NSAIDs. Members of this family of drugs should not be used during the third trimester of pregnancy (last 12 weeks) unless specifically prescribed by a clinician. See the Appendix for "Non-Steroidal, Anti-Inflammatory Drugs (NSAIDs) in Pregnancy," which describes the serious problems these drugs may cause for unborn babies when taken in the third trimester of pregnancy.

2. Women attempting to conceive should not use any NSAID, including aspirin, because of the findings in animals that these drugs may block implantation of the early embryo in the wall of the uterus, in effect preventing pregnancy.

Remember: All pregnancies have a background risk of 3% or more for a serious birth defect, even when mom doesn't take a drug of any kind. If you are pregnant or planning a pregnancy, always let your healthcare provider know before taking any drug, prescription or non-prescription, or herbal remedy.

Excedrin® Migraine Pain Reliever Caplets

Active Ingredient:	Pregnancy Risk Category:
Acetaminophen	B
Caffeine	B
Aspirin	Aspirin has two pregnancy risk categories: **C** when used in the first or second trimesters of pregnancy; **D** if used in the third trimester. (See Helpful Hints on the next page.)

Helpful Hints and Reminders: Each pregnancy risk category (**A**, **B**, **C**, **D**, or **X**) is explained on the last page of this section.

1. Aspirin is a member of the non-steroidal, anti-inflammatory family of drugs, or NSAIDs. Members of this family of drugs should not be used during the third trimester of pregnancy (last 12 weeks) unless specifically prescribed by a clinician. See the Appendix for "Non-Steroidal, Anti-Inflammatory Drugs (NSAIDs) in Pregnancy," which describes the serious problems these drugs may cause for unborn babies when taken in the third trimester of pregnancy.

2. Women attempting to conceive should not use any NSAID, including aspirin, because of the findings in animals that these drugs may block implantation of the early embryo in the wall of the uterus, in effect preventing pregnancy.

Remember: All pregnancies have a background risk of 3% or more for a serious birth defect, even when mom doesn't take a drug of any kind. If you are pregnant or planning a pregnancy, always let your healthcare provider know before taking any drug, prescription or non-prescription, or herbal remedy.

Excedrin® PM Caplets & Tablets

Active Ingredient:	Pregnancy Risk Category:
Acetaminophen	B
Diphenhydramine citrate	B

Helpful Hints and Reminders: Each pregnancy risk category (**A**, **B**, **C**, **D**, or **X**) is explained on the last page of this section.

Remember: All pregnancies have a background risk of 3% or more for a serious birth defect, even when mom doesn't take a drug of any kind. If you are pregnant or planning a pregnancy, always let your healthcare provider know before taking any drug, prescription or non-prescription, or herbal remedy.

Excedrin® Tension Headache Geltabs, Tablets, and Caplets

Active Ingredient:	Pregnancy Risk Category:
Acetaminophen	B
Caffeine	B

Helpful Hints and Reminders: Each pregnancy risk category (**A**, **B**, **C**, **D**, or **X**) is explained on the last page of this section.

Remember: All pregnancies have a background risk of 3% or more for a serious birth defect, even when mom doesn't take a drug of any kind. If you are pregnant or planning a pregnancy, always let your healthcare provider know before taking any drug, prescription or non-prescription, or herbal remedy.

Goody's® Body Pain

Active Ingredient:	Pregnancy Risk Category:
Acetaminophen	B
Aspirin	Aspirin has two pregnancy risk categories: **C** when used in the first or second trimesters of pregnancy; **D** if used in the third trimester. (See Helpful Hints below.)

Helpful Hints and Reminders: Each pregnancy risk category (**A**, **B**, **C**, **D**, or **X**) is explained on the last page of this section.

1. Aspirin is a member of the non-steroidal, anti-inflammatory family of drugs, or NSAIDs. Members of this family of drugs should not be used during the third trimester of pregnancy (last 12 weeks) unless specifically prescribed by a clinician. See the Appendix for "Non-Steroidal, Anti-Inflammatory Drugs (NSAIDs) in Pregnancy," which describes the serious problems these drugs may cause for unborn babies when taken in the third trimester of pregnancy.

2. Women attempting to conceive should not use any NSAID, including aspirin, because of the findings in animals that these drugs may block implantation of the early embryo in the wall of the uterus, in effect preventing pregnancy.

Remember: All pregnancies have a background risk of 3% or more for a serious birth defect, even when mom doesn't take a drug of any kind. If you are pregnant or planning a pregnancy, always let your healthcare provider know before taking any drug, prescription or non-prescription, or herbal remedy.

Goody's® Cool Orange

Active Ingredient:	Pregnancy Risk Category:
Acetaminophen	B
Caffeine	B
Aspirin	Aspirin has two pregnancy risk categories: **C** when used in the first or second trimesters of pregnancy; **D** if used in the third trimester. (See Helpful Hints below.)

Helpful Hints and Reminders: Each pregnancy risk category (**A**, **B**, **C**, **D**, or **X**) is explained on the last page of this section.

1. Aspirin is a member of the non-steroidal, anti-inflammatory family of drugs, or NSAIDs. Members of this family of drugs should not be used during the third trimester of pregnancy (last 12 weeks) unless specifically prescribed by a clinician. See the Appendix for "Non-Steroidal, Anti-Inflammatory Drugs (NSAIDs) in Pregnancy," which describes the serious problems these drugs may cause for unborn babies when taken in the third trimester of pregnancy.

2. Women attempting to conceive should not use any NSAID, including aspirin, because of the findings in animals that these drugs may block implantation of the early embryo in the wall of the uterus, in effect preventing pregnancy.

Remember: All pregnancies have a background risk of 3% or more for a serious birth defect, even when mom doesn't take a drug of any kind. If you are pregnant or planning a pregnancy, always let your healthcare provider know before taking any drug, prescription or non-prescription, or herbal remedy.

Goody's® Extra Strength

Active Ingredient:	Pregnancy Risk Category:
Acetaminophen	B
Caffeine	B
Aspirin	Aspirin has two pregnancy risk categories: **C** when used in the first or second trimesters of pregnancy; **D** if used in the third trimester. (See Helpful Hints below.)

Helpful Hints and Reminders: Each pregnancy risk category (**A**, **B**, **C**, **D**, or **X**) is explained on the last page of this section.

1. Aspirin is a member of the non-steroidal, anti-inflammatory family of drugs, or NSAIDs. Members of this family of drugs should not be used during the third trimester of pregnancy (last 12 weeks) unless specifically prescribed by a clinician. See the Appendix for "Non-Steroidal, Anti-Inflammatory Drugs (NSAIDs) in Pregnancy," which describes the serious problems these drugs may cause for unborn babies when taken in the third trimester of pregnancy.

2. Women attempting to conceive should not use any NSAID, including aspirin, because of the findings in animals that these drugs may block implantation of the early embryo in the wall of the uterus, in effect preventing pregnancy.

Remember: All pregnancies have a background risk of 3% or more for a serious birth defect, even when mom doesn't take a drug of any kind. If you are pregnant or planning a pregnancy, always let your healthcare provider know before taking any drug, prescription or non-prescription, or herbal remedy.

Goody's® PM

Active Ingredient:	Pregnancy Risk Category:
Acetaminophen	B
Diphenhydramine citrate	B

Helpful Hints and Reminders: Each pregnancy risk category (**A**, **B**, **C**, **D**, or **X**) is explained on the last page of this section.

Remember: All pregnancies have a background risk of 3% or more for a serious birth defect, even when mom doesn't take a drug of any kind. If you are pregnant or planning a pregnancy, always let your healthcare provider know before taking any drug, prescription or non-prescription, or herbal remedy.

Kirkland Signature™ Ibuprofen 200 Mg Tablets

Active Ingredient:	Pregnancy Risk Category:
Ibuprofen	Ibuprofen has two pregnancy risk categories: **B** when used in the first or second trimesters of pregnancy; **D** if used in the third trimester. (See Helpful Hints below.)

Helpful Hints and Reminders: Each pregnancy risk category (**A**, **B**, **C**, **D**, or **X**) is explained on the last page of this section.

1. Ibuprofen is a member of the non-steroidal, anti-inflammatory family of drugs, or NSAIDs. Members of this family of drugs should not be used during the third trimester of pregnancy (last 12 weeks) unless specifically prescribed by a clinician. See the Appendix for "Non-Steroidal, Anti-Inflammatory Drugs (NSAIDs) in Pregnancy," which describes the serious problems these drugs may cause for unborn babies when taken in the third trimester of pregnancy.

2. Women attempting to conceive should not use any NSAID, including ibuprofen, because of the findings in animals that these drugs may block implantation of the early embryo in the wall of the uterus, in effect preventing pregnancy.

Remember: All pregnancies have a background risk of 3% or more for a serious birth defect, even when mom doesn't take a drug of any kind. If you are pregnant or planning a pregnancy, always let your healthcare provider know before taking any drug, prescription or non-prescription, or herbal remedy.

Kirkland Signature™ Naproxen Sodium 220 Mg

Active Ingredient:	Pregnancy Risk Category:
Naproxen sodium	Naproxen sodium has two pregnancy risk categories: **C** when used in the first or second trimesters of pregnancy; **D** if used in the third trimester. (See Helpful Hints below.)

Helpful Hints and Reminders: Each pregnancy risk category (**A**, **B**, **C**, **D**, or **X**) is explained on the last page of this section.

1. Naproxen sodium is a member of the non-steroidal, anti-inflammatory family of drugs, or NSAIDs. Members of this family of drugs should not be used during the third trimester of pregnancy (last 12 weeks) unless specifically prescribed by a clinician. See the Appendix for "Non-Steroidal, Anti-Inflammatory Drugs (NSAIDs) in Pregnancy," which describes the serious problems these drugs may cause for unborn babies when taken in the third trimester of pregnancy.

2. Women attempting to conceive should not use any NSAID, including naproxen sodium, because of the findings in animals that these drugs may block implantation of the early embryo in the wall of the uterus, in effect preventing pregnancy.

Remember: All pregnancies have a background risk of 3% or more for a serious birth defect, even when mom doesn't take a drug of any kind. If you are pregnant or planning a pregnancy, always let your healthcare provider know before taking any drug, prescription or non-prescription, or herbal remedy.

Motrin® IB Caplets & Tablets

Active Ingredient:	Pregnancy Risk Category:
Ibuprofen	Ibuprofen has two pregnancy risk categories: **B** when used in the first or second trimesters of pregnancy; **D** if used in the third trimester. (See Helpful Hints below.)

Helpful Hints and Reminders: Each pregnancy risk category (**A**, **B**, **C**, **D**, or **X**) is explained on the last page of this section.

1. Ibuprofen is a member of the non-steroidal, anti-inflammatory family of drugs, or NSAIDs. Members of this family of drugs should not be used during the third trimester of pregnancy (last 12 weeks) unless specifically prescribed by a clinician. See the Appendix for "Non-Steroidal, Anti-Inflammatory Drugs (NSAIDs) in Pregnancy," which describes the serious problems these drugs may cause for unborn babies when taken in the third trimester of pregnancy.

2. Women attempting to conceive should not use any NSAID, including ibuprofen, because of the findings in animals that these drugs may block implantation of the early embryo in the wall of the uterus, in effect preventing pregnancy.

Remember: All pregnancies have a background risk of 3% or more for a serious birth defect, even when mom doesn't take a drug of any kind. If you are pregnant or planning a pregnancy, always let your healthcare provider know before taking any drug, prescription or non-prescription, or herbal remedy.

Motrin® PM Caplets

Active Ingredient:	Pregnancy Risk Category:
Diphenhydramine citrate	B

(*continued*)

Ibuprofen	Ibuprofen has two pregnancy risk categories: **B** when used in the first or second trimesters of pregnancy; **D** if used in the third trimester. (See Helpful Hints below.)

Helpful Hints and Reminders: Each pregnancy risk category (**A**, **B**, **C**, **D**, or **X**) is explained on the last page of this section.

1. Ibuprofen is a member of the non-steroidal, anti-inflammatory family of drugs, or NSAIDs. Members of this family of drugs should not be used during the third trimester of pregnancy (last 12 weeks) unless specifically prescribed by a clinician. See the Appendix for "Non-Steroidal, Anti-Inflammatory Drugs (NSAIDs) in Pregnancy," which describes the serious problems these drugs may cause for unborn babies when taken in the third trimester of pregnancy.

2. Women attempting to conceive should not use any NSAID, including ibuprofen, because of the findings in animals that these drugs may block implantation of the early embryo in the wall of the uterus, in effect preventing pregnancy.

Remember: All pregnancies have a background risk of 3% or more for a serious birth defect, even when mom doesn't take a drug of any kind. If you are pregnant or planning a pregnancy, always let your healthcare provider know before taking any drug, prescription or non-prescription, or herbal remedy.

Rite Aid® Acetaminophen Extended-Release Pain Reliever Tablets

Active Ingredient:	Pregnancy Risk Category:
Acetaminophen	B

Helpful Hints and Reminders: Each pregnancy risk category (**A**, **B**, **C**, **D**, or **X**) is explained on the last page of this section.

Remember: All pregnancies have a background risk of 3% or more for a serious birth defect, even when mom doesn't take a drug of any kind. If you are pregnant or planning a pregnancy, always let your healthcare provider know before taking any drug, prescription or non-prescription, or herbal remedy.

Rite Aid® Ibuprofen, 200 Mg Coated Tablets

Active Ingredient:	Pregnancy Risk Category:
Ibuprofen	Ibuprofen has two pregnancy risk categories: **B** when used in the first or second trimesters of pregnancy; **D** if used in the third trimester. (See Helpful Hints below.)

Helpful Hints and Reminders: Each pregnancy risk category (**A**, **B**, **C**, **D**, or **X**) is explained on the last page of this section.

1. Ibuprofen is a member of the non-steroidal, anti-inflammatory family of drugs, or NSAIDs. Members of this family of drugs should not be used during the third trimester of pregnancy (last 12 weeks) unless specifically prescribed by a clinician. See the Appendix for "Non-Steroidal, Anti-Inflammatory Drugs (NSAIDs) in Pregnancy," which describes the serious problems these drugs may cause for unborn babies when taken in the third trimester of pregnancy.

2. Women attempting to conceive should not use any NSAID, including ibuprofen, because of the findings in animals that these drugs may block implantation of the early embryo in the wall of the uterus, in effect preventing pregnancy.

Remember: All pregnancies have a background risk of 3% or more for a serious birth defect, even when mom doesn't take a drug of any kind. If you are pregnant or planning a pregnancy, always let your healthcare provider know before taking any drug, prescription or non-prescription, or herbal remedy.

St. Joseph® 81 Mg Aspirin Enteric Safety-Coated Tablets

Active Ingredient:	Pregnancy Risk Category:
Aspirin	Aspirin has two pregnancy risk categories: **C** when used in the first or second trimesters of pregnancy; **D** if used in the third trimester. (See Helpful Hints below.)

Helpful Hints and Reminders: Each pregnancy risk category (**A**, **B**, **C**, **D**, or **X**) is explained on the last page of this section.

1. Aspirin is a member of the non-steroidal, anti-inflammatory family of drugs, or NSAIDs. Members of this family of drugs should not be used during the third trimester of pregnancy (last 12 weeks) unless specifically prescribed by a clinician. See the Appendix for "Non-Steroidal, Anti-Inflammatory Drugs (NSAIDs) in Pregnancy," which describes the serious problems these drugs may cause for unborn babies when taken in the third trimester of pregnancy.

2. Women attempting to conceive should not use any NSAID, including aspirin, because of the findings in animals that these drugs may block implantation of the early embryo in the wall of the uterus, in effect preventing pregnancy.

Remember: All pregnancies have a background risk of 3% or more for a serious birth defect, even when mom doesn't take a drug of any kind. If you are pregnant or planning a pregnancy, always let your healthcare provider know before taking any drug, prescription or non-prescription, or herbal remedy.

St. Joseph® 81 Mg Chewable Aspirin

Active Ingredient:	Pregnancy Risk Category:
Aspirin	Aspirin has two pregnancy risk categories: **C** when used in the first or second trimesters of pregnancy; **D** if used in the third trimester. (See Helpful Hints on the next page.)

Helpful Hints and Reminders: Each pregnancy risk category (**A**, **B**, **C**, **D**, or **X**) is explained on the last page of this section.

1. Aspirin is a member of the non-steroidal, anti-inflammatory family of drugs, or NSAIDs. Members of this family of drugs should not be used during the third trimester of pregnancy (last 12 weeks) unless specifically prescribed by a clinician. See the Appendix for "Non-Steroidal, Anti-Inflammatory Drugs (NSAIDs) in Pregnancy," which describes the serious problems these drugs may cause for unborn babies when taken in the third trimester of pregnancy.

2. Women attempting to conceive should not use any NSAID, including aspirin, because of the findings in animals that these drugs may block implantation of the early embryo in the wall of the uterus, in effect preventing pregnancy.

Remember: All pregnancies have a background risk of 3% or more for a serious birth defect, even when mom doesn't take a drug of any kind. If you are pregnant or planning a pregnancy, always let your healthcare provider know before taking any drug, prescription or non-prescription, or herbal remedy.

Target® Acetaminophen Pain Relief Caplets

Active Ingredient:	Pregnancy Risk Category:
Acetaminophen	B

Helpful Hints and Reminders: Each pregnancy risk category (**A**, **B**, **C**, **D**, or **X**) is explained on the last page of this section.

Remember: All pregnancies have a background risk of 3% or more for a serious birth defect, even when mom doesn't take a drug of any kind. If you are pregnant or planning a pregnancy, always let your healthcare provider know before taking any drug, prescription or non-prescription, or herbal remedy.

Target® Extra Strength Pain Reliever PM Caplets

Active Ingredient:	Pregnancy Risk Category:
Acetaminophen	B
Diphenhydramine Hcl	B

Helpful Hints and Reminders: Each pregnancy risk category (**A**, **B**, **C**, **D**, or **X**) is explained on the last page of this section.

Remember: All pregnancies have a background risk of 3% or more for a serious birth defect, even when mom doesn't take a drug of any kind. If you are pregnant or planning a pregnancy, always let your healthcare provider know before taking any drug, prescription or non-prescription, or herbal remedy.

Target® Migraine Formula Caplets

Active Ingredient:	Pregnancy Risk Category:
Acetaminophen	B
Caffeine	B
Aspirin	Aspirin has two pregnancy risk categories: **C** when used in the first or second trimesters of pregnancy; **D** if used in the third trimester. (See Helpful Hints below.)

Helpful Hints and Reminders: Each pregnancy risk category (**A**, **B**, **C**, **D**, or **X**) is explained on the last page of this section.

1. Aspirin is a member of the non-steroidal, anti-inflammatory family of drugs, or NSAIDs. Members of this family of drugs should not be used during the third trimester of pregnancy (last 12 weeks) unless specifically prescribed by a clinician. See

the Appendix for "Non-Steroidal, Anti-Inflammatory Drugs (NSAIDs) in Pregnancy," which describes the serious problems these drugs may cause for unborn babies when taken in the third trimester of pregnancy.

2. Women attempting to conceive should not use any NSAID, including aspirin, because of the findings in animals that these drugs may block implantation of the early embryo in the wall of the uterus, in effect preventing pregnancy.

Remember: All pregnancies have a background risk of 3% or more for a serious birth defect, even when mom doesn't take a drug of any kind. If you are pregnant or planning a pregnancy, always let your healthcare provider know before taking any drug, prescription or non-prescription, or herbal remedy.

Target® Naproxen Sodium Caplets

Active Ingredient:	Pregnancy Risk Category:
Naproxen sodium	Naproxen sodium has two pregnancy risk categories: **C** when used in the first or second trimesters of pregnancy; **D** if used in the third trimester. (See Helpful Hints below.)

Helpful Hints and Reminders: Each pregnancy risk category (**A**, **B**, **C**, **D**, or **X**) is explained on the last page of this section.

1. Naproxen sodium is a member of the non-steroidal, anti-inflammatory family of drugs, or NSAIDs. Members of this family of drugs should not be used during the third trimester of pregnancy (last 12 weeks) unless specifically prescribed by a clinician. See the Appendix for "Non-Steroidal, Anti-Inflammatory Drugs (NSAIDs) in Pregnancy," which describes the serious problems these drugs may cause for unborn babies when taken in the third trimester of pregnancy.

Tylenol® Arthritis Pain

2. Women attempting to conceive should not use any NSAID, including naproxen sodium, because of the findings in animals that these drugs may block implantation of the early embryo in the wall of the uterus, in effect preventing pregnancy.

Remember: All pregnancies have a background risk of 3% or more for a serious birth defect, even when mom doesn't take a drug of any kind. If you are pregnant or planning a pregnancy, always let your healthcare provider know before taking any drug, prescription or non-prescription, or herbal remedy.

Tylenol® 8 Hour

Active Ingredient:	Pregnancy Risk Category:
Acetaminophen	B

Helpful Hints and Reminders: Each pregnancy risk category (**A**, **B**, **C**, **D**, or **X**) is explained on the last page of this section.

Remember: All pregnancies have a background risk of 3% or more for a serious birth defect, even when mom doesn't take a drug of any kind. If you are pregnant or planning a pregnancy, always let your healthcare provider know before taking any drug, prescription or non-prescription, or herbal remedy.

Tylenol® Arthritis Pain

Active Ingredient:	Pregnancy Risk Category:
Acetaminophen	B

Helpful Hints and Reminders: Each pregnancy risk category (**A**, **B**, **C**, **D**, or **X**) is explained on the last page of this section.

Remember: All pregnancies have a background risk of 3% or more for a serious birth defect, even when mom doesn't take a drug of any kind. If you are pregnant or planning a pregnancy, always let your healthcare provider know before taking any drug, prescription or non-prescription, or herbal remedy.

Tylenol® Extra Strength

Active Ingredient:	Pregnancy Risk Category:
Acetaminophen	B

Helpful Hints and Reminders: Each pregnancy risk category (**A**, **B**, **C**, **D**, or **X**) is explained on the last page of this section.

Remember: All pregnancies have a background risk of 3% or more for a serious birth defect, even when mom doesn't take a drug of any kind. If you are pregnant or planning a pregnancy, always let your healthcare provider know before taking any drug, prescription or non-prescription, or herbal remedy.

Tylenol® PM

Active Ingredient:	Pregnancy Risk Category:
Acetaminophen	B
Diphenhydramine Hcl	B

Helpful Hints and Reminders: Each pregnancy risk category (**A**, **B**, **C**, **D**, or **X**) is explained on the last page of this section.

Remember: All pregnancies have a background risk of 3% or more for a serious birth defect, even when mom doesn't take a drug of any kind. If you are pregnant or planning a pregnancy, always let your healthcare provider know before taking any drug, prescription or non-prescription, or herbal remedy.

Tylenol® Regular Strength

Active Ingredient:	Pregnancy Risk Category:
Acetaminophen	B

Helpful Hints and Reminders: Each pregnancy risk category (**A**, **B**, **C**, **D**, or **X**) is explained on the last page of this section.

Remember: All pregnancies have a background risk of 3% or more for a serious birth defect, even when mom doesn't take a drug of any kind.

If you are pregnant or planning a pregnancy, always let your healthcare provider know before taking any drug, prescription or non-prescription, or herbal remedy.

Unisom® PM Pain SleepCaps

Active Ingredient:	Pregnancy Risk Category:
Diphenhydramine Hcl	B
Acetaminophen	B

Helpful Hints and Reminders: Each pregnancy risk category (**A**, **B**, **C**, **D**, or **X**) is explained on the last page of this section.

Remember: All pregnancies have a background risk of 3% or more for a serious birth defect, even when mom doesn't take a drug of any kind. If you are pregnant or planning a pregnancy, always let your healthcare provider know before taking any drug, prescription or non-prescription, or herbal remedy.

Up & Up™ Ibuprofen Pain Relief 200 Mg

Active Ingredient:	Pregnancy Risk Category:
Ibuprofen	Ibuprofen has two pregnancy risk categories: **B** when used in the first or second trimesters of pregnancy; **D** if used in the third trimester. (See Helpful Hints below.)

Helpful Hints and Reminders: Each pregnancy risk category (**A**, **B**, **C**, **D**, or **X**) is explained on the last page of this section.

1. Ibuprofen is a member of the non-steroidal, anti-inflammatory family of drugs, or NSAIDs. Members of this family of drugs should not be used during the third trimester of pregnancy (last 12 weeks) unless specifically prescribed by a clinician. See the Appendix for "Non-Steroidal, Anti-Inflammatory Drugs (NSAIDs) in Pregnancy," which describes the serious problems

these drugs may cause for unborn babies when taken in the third trimester of pregnancy.

2. Women attempting to conceive should not use any NSAID, including ibuprofen, because of the findings in animals that these drugs may block implantation of the early embryo in the wall of the uterus, in effect preventing pregnancy.

Remember: All pregnancies have a background risk of 3% or more for a serious birth defect, even when mom doesn't take a drug of any kind. If you are pregnant or planning a pregnancy, always let your healthcare provider know before taking any drug, prescription or non-prescription, or herbal remedy.

Vicks® Formula 44® Custom Care™ Body Aches

Active Ingredient:	Pregnancy Risk Category:
Acetaminophen	B

Helpful Hints and Reminders: Each pregnancy risk category (**A**, **B**, **C**, **D**, or **X**) is explained on the last page of this section.

Remember: All pregnancies have a background risk of 3% or more for a serious birth defect, even when mom doesn't take a drug of any kind. If you are pregnant or planning a pregnancy, always let your healthcare provider know before taking any drug, prescription or non-prescription, or herbal remedy.

Vicks® Formula 44® Custom Care™ Sore Throat Lozenges

Active Ingredient:	Pregnancy Risk Category:
Benzocaine	C
Menthol	**Risk is undetermined.** The FDA has not assigned a pregnancy risk category to menthol. (See Helpful Hint on the next page.)

Helpful Hints and Reminders: Each pregnancy risk category (**A**, **B**, **C**, **D**, or **X**) is explained on the last page of this section.

1. Menthol is a common ingredient in many throat lozenges and sprays. There are no studies using the drug in pregnant animals or pregnant women. However, the risk of adverse fetal effects is believed to be quite small, according to the Illinois Teratogen Information Service (ITIS).

Remember: All pregnancies have a background risk of 3% or more for a serious birth defect, even when mom doesn't take a drug of any kind. If you are pregnant or planning a pregnancy, always let your healthcare provider know before taking any drug, prescription or non-prescription, or herbal remedy.

Vicks® Formula 44® Custom Care™ Sore Throat Spray

Active Ingredient:	Pregnancy Risk Category:
Glycerin	C
Phenol	**Risk is undetermined.** The FDA has not assigned a pregnancy risk category to this active ingredient. (See Helpful Hint below.)

Helpful Hints and Reminders: Each pregnancy risk category (**A**, **B**, **C**, **D**, or **X**) is explained on the last page of this section.

1. The limited amount of information about exposure to phenol in pregnancy indicates that it is not associated with either an increased incidence of birth defects or miscarriages at concentrations that are not toxic to mom.

Remember: All pregnancies have a background risk of 3% or more for a serious birth defect, even when mom doesn't take a drug of any kind. If you are pregnant or planning a pregnancy, always let your healthcare provider know before taking any drug, prescription or non-prescription, or herbal remedy.

Walgreens® Low Dose Aspirin Safety Coated Tablets

Active Ingredient:	Pregnancy Risk Category:
Aspirin	Aspirin has two pregnancy risk categories: **C** when used in the first or second trimesters of pregnancy; **D** if used in the third trimester. (See Helpful Hints below.)

Helpful Hints and Reminders: Each pregnancy risk category (**A**, **B**, **C**, **D**, or **X**) is explained on the last page of this section.

1. Aspirin is a member of the non-steroidal, anti-inflammatory family of drugs, or NSAIDs. Members of this family of drugs should not be used during the third trimester of pregnancy (last 12 weeks) unless specifically prescribed by a clinician. See the Appendix for "Non-Steroidal, Anti-Inflammatory Drugs (NSAIDs) in Pregnancy," which describes the serious problems these drugs may cause for unborn babies when taken in the third trimester of pregnancy.

2. Women attempting to conceive should not use any NSAID, including aspirin, because of the findings in animals that these drugs may block implantation of the early embryo in the wall of the uterus, in effect preventing pregnancy.

Remember: All pregnancies have a background risk of 3% or more for a serious birth defect, even when mom doesn't take a drug of any kind. If you are pregnant or planning a pregnancy, always let your healthcare provider know before taking any drug, prescription or non-prescription, or herbal remedy.

The FDA's Pregnancy Risk Categories: A, B, C, D, X

Adapted to the Active Ingredients in Nonprescription drugs

Category A: Controlled studies using the active ingredient in pregnant women have not shown harmful fetal effects throughout pregnancy, and the possibility of fetal harm seems remote. My comment: *Though apparently safe, these active ingredients should still only be used in pregnancy when clearly indicated.*

Category B: Either studies have shown no evidence of fetal harm when using the active ingredient in pregnant animals, but no controlled studies have been done in pregnant women, **or** studies have shown evidence of fetal harm when using the active ingredient in pregnant animals, but controlled studies in pregnant women have not shown evidence of fetal harm. My comment: *These active ingredients should only be used in pregnancy when clearly indicated.*

Category C: Either studies have shown evidence of fetal harm when using the active ingredient in pregnant animals, but no controlled studies have been done in pregnant women, **or** studies using the active ingredient in pregnant animals have not been done, and studies of pregnant women are insufficient to reach a conclusion. These active ingredients should only be used by a pregnant woman if the potential benefit justifies the potential risk of fetal harm, which, in many cases, is unknown. My comment: *It's impossible to calculate the potential risk of fetal harm when, in many cases, it's unknown. Thus, these active ingredients should only be used in pregnancy when clearly needed.*

Category D: Studies have shown evidence of fetal harm when using the active ingredient in pregnant women. However, the potential benefit of using the active ingredient in some life-threatening situations for mom may outweigh the potential risk of fetal harm. For example, when mom requires cancer treatment or when she has a serious disease for which safer active ingredients cannot be used or are less effective. My comment: *These exceptional indications rarely occur when considering a nonprescription drug in pregnancy.*

Category X: My comment: *Because the risk of fetal harm is too high, no Category X active ingredients have been approved for use in nonprescription drugs.*

Active Ingredients Assigned Two Pregnancy Risk Categories: Some active ingredients have two pregnancy risk categories, depending on which trimester of pregnancy the active ingredient is used. For example, naproxen sodium, the active ingredient in Aleve, belongs to Category **B** when used in the first and second trimesters of pregnancy. If used in the third trimester, however, the active ingredient belongs to Category **D**. My comment: *This means naproxen sodium should not be used in the third trimester unless prescribed by a physician who has advised her patient of the risks involved.*

Section 11: Skin Disorders

Aveeno® Maximum Strength Anti-Itch Cream, 1% Hydrocortisone

Active Ingredient:	Pregnancy Risk Category:
Hydrocortisone 1%	Hydrocortisone has two pregnancy risk categories: **C** when used in the second or third trimesters of pregnancy; **D** if used in the first trimester.

Helpful Hints and Reminders: Each pregnancy risk category (**A**, **B**, **C**, **D**, or **X**) is explained on the last page of this section.

1. Topical corticosteroids should be used in pregnancy only if the potential benefit for mom outweighs the potential risk to her fetus. This class of drug should not be used extensively in pregnant women, in large amounts or for extensive periods of time, especially during the first trimester.

Remember: All pregnancies have a background risk of 3% or more for a serious birth defect, even when mom doesn't take a drug of any kind. If you are pregnant or planning a pregnancy, always let your healthcare provider know before taking any drug, prescription or non-prescription, or herbal remedy.

Benadryl® Extra Strength Itch Relief Stick

Active Ingredient:	Pregnancy Risk Category:
Diphenhydramine Hcl	B
Zinc acetate	A

Helpful Hints and Reminders: Each pregnancy risk category (**A**, **B**, **C**, **D**, or **X**) is explained on the last page of this section.

Remember: All pregnancies have a background risk of 3% or more for a serious birth defect, even when mom doesn't take a drug of any kind. If you are pregnant or planning a pregnancy, always let your healthcare provider know before taking any drug, prescription or non-prescription, or herbal remedy.

Benadryl® Extra Strength Itch Stopping Cream

Active Ingredient:	Pregnancy Risk Category:
Diphenhydramine Hcl	B
Zinc acetate	A

Helpful Hints and Reminders: Each pregnancy risk category (**A**, **B**, **C**, **D**, or **X**) is explained on the last page of this section.

Remember: All pregnancies have a background risk of 3% or more for a serious birth defect, even when mom doesn't take a drug of any kind. If you are pregnant or planning a pregnancy, always let your healthcare provider know before taking any drug, prescription or non-prescription, or herbal remedy.

Benadryl® Extra Strength Spray

Active Ingredient:	Pregnancy Risk Category:
Diphenhydramine Hcl	B
Zinc acetate	A

Helpful Hints and Reminders: Each pregnancy risk category (**A**, **B**, **C**, **D**, or **X**) is explained on the last page of this section.

Remember: All pregnancies have a background risk of 3% or more for a serious birth defect, even when mom doesn't take a drug of any kind. If you are pregnant or planning a pregnancy, always let your healthcare provider know before taking any drug, prescription or non-prescription, or herbal remedy.

Benadryl® Original Strength Itch Stopping Cream

Active Ingredient:	Pregnancy Risk Category:
Diphenhydramine Hcl	B
Zinc acetate	A

Helpful Hints and Reminders: Each pregnancy risk category (**A**, **B**, **C**, **D**, or **X**) is explained on the last page of this section.

Remember: All pregnancies have a background risk of 3% or more for a serious birth defect, even when mom doesn't take a drug of any kind. If you are pregnant or planning a pregnancy, always let your healthcare provider know before taking any drug, prescription or non-prescription, or herbal remedy.

Benadryl® Readymist Itch Stopping Spray

Active Ingredient:	Pregnancy Risk Category:
Diphenhydramine Hcl	B
Zinc acetate	A

Helpful Hints and Reminders: Each pregnancy risk category (**A**, **B**, **C**, **D**, or **X**) is explained on the last page of this section.

Remember: All pregnancies have a background risk of 3% or more for a serious birth defect, even when mom doesn't take a drug of any kind. If you are pregnant or planning a pregnancy, always let your healthcare provider know before taking any drug, prescription or non-prescription, or herbal remedy.

Cortaid® Advanced 12 Hour Anti-Itch Cream

Active Ingredient:	Pregnancy Risk Category:
Hydrocortisone	Hydrocortisone has two pregnancy risk categories: **C** when used in the second or third trimesters of pregnancy; **D** if used in the first trimester.

Helpful Hints and Reminders: Each pregnancy risk category (**A**, **B**, **C**, **D**, or **X**) is explained on the last page of this section.

1. Topical corticosteroids should be used in pregnancy only if the potential benefit for mom outweighs the potential risk to her fetus. This class of drug should not be used extensively in pregnant women, in large amounts or for extensive periods of time, especially during the first trimester.

Remember: All pregnancies have a background risk of 3% or more for a serious birth defect, even when mom doesn't take a drug of any kind. If you are pregnant or planning a pregnancy, always let your healthcare provider know before taking any drug, prescription or non-prescription, or herbal remedy.

Cortaid® Intensive Therapy Cooling Spray

Active Ingredient:	Pregnancy Risk Category:
Hydrocortisone	Hydrocortisone has two pregnancy risk categories: **C** when used in the second or third trimesters of pregnancy; **D** if used in the first trimester.

Helpful Hints and Reminders: Each pregnancy risk category (**A**, **B**, **C**, **D**, or **X**) is explained on the last page of this section.

1. Topical corticosteroids should be used in pregnancy only if the potential benefit for mom outweighs the potential risk to her fetus. This class of drug should not be used extensively in

Cortaid® Intensive Therapy Moisturizing Cream **261**

pregnant women, in large amounts or for extensive periods of time, especially during the first trimester.

Remember: All pregnancies have a background risk of 3% or more for a serious birth defect, even when mom doesn't take a drug of any kind. If you are pregnant or planning a pregnancy, always let your healthcare provider know before taking any drug, prescription or non-prescription, or herbal remedy.

Cortaid® Intensive Therapy Moisturizing Cream

Active Ingredient:	Pregnancy Risk Category:
Hydrocortisone	Hydrocortisone has two pregnancy risk categories: **C** when used in the second or third trimesters of pregnancy; **D** if used in the first trimester.

Helpful Hints and Reminders: Each pregnancy risk category (**A**, **B**, **C**, **D**, or **X**) is explained on the last page of this section.

1. Topical corticosteroids should be used in pregnancy only if the potential benefit for mom outweighs the potential risk to her fetus. This class of drug should not be used extensively in pregnant women, in large amounts or for extensive periods of time, especially during the first trimester.

Remember: All pregnancies have a background risk of 3% or more for a serious birth defect, even when mom doesn't take a drug of any kind. If you are pregnant or planning a pregnancy, always let your healthcare provider know before taking any drug, prescription or non-prescription, or herbal remedy.

Cortaid® Maximum Strength Cream

Active Ingredient:	Pregnancy Risk Category:
Hydrocortisone	Hydrocortisone has two pregnancy risk categories: **C** when used in the second or third trimesters of pregnancy; **D** if used in the first trimester.

Helpful Hints and Reminders: Each pregnancy risk category (**A**, **B**, **C**, **D**, or **X**) is explained on the last page of this section.

1. Topical corticosteroids should be used in pregnancy only if the potential benefit for mom outweighs the potential risk to her fetus. This class of drug should not be used extensively in pregnant women, in large amounts or for extensive periods of time, especially during the first trimester.

Remember: All pregnancies have a background risk of 3% or more for a serious birth defect, even when mom doesn't take a drug of any kind. If you are pregnant or planning a pregnancy, always let your healthcare provider know before taking any drug, prescription or non-prescription, or herbal remedy.

Cortaid® Maximum Strength Ointment

Active Ingredient:	Pregnancy Risk Category:
Hydrocortisone	Hydrocortisone has two pregnancy risk categories: **C** when used in the second or third trimesters of pregnancy; **D** if used in the first trimester.

Helpful Hints and Reminders: Each pregnancy risk category (**A**, **B**, **C**, **D**, or **X**) is explained on the last page of this section.

1. Topical corticosteroids should be used in pregnancy only if the potential benefit for mom outweighs the potential risk to her fetus. This class of drug should not be used extensively in

pregnant women, in large amounts or for extensive periods of time, especially during the first trimester.

Remember: All pregnancies have a background risk of 3% or more for a serious birth defect, even when mom doesn't take a drug of any kind. If you are pregnant or planning a pregnancy, always let your healthcare provider know before taking any drug, prescription or non-prescription, or herbal remedy.

Dermarest® Eczema Medicated Lotion

Active Ingredient:	Pregnancy Risk Category:
Hydrocortisone 1%	Hydrocortisone has two pregnancy risk categories: **C** when used in the second or third trimesters of pregnancy; **D** if used in the first trimester. (See Helpful Hints below.)

Helpful Hints and Reminders: Each pregnancy risk category (**A**, **B**, **C**, **D**, or **X**) is explained on the last page of this section.

1. Topical corticosteroids should be used in pregnancy only if the potential benefit for mom outweighs the potential risk to her fetus. This class of drug should not be used extensively in pregnant women, in large amounts or for extensive periods of time, especially during the first trimester.

Remember: All pregnancies have a background risk of 3% or more for a serious birth defect, even when mom doesn't take a drug of any kind. If you are pregnant or planning a pregnancy, always let your healthcare provider know before taking any drug, prescription or non-prescription, or herbal remedy.

Dermarest® Psoriasis Medicated Skin Treatment

Active Ingredient:	Pregnancy Risk Category:
Salicylic acid 3%	**C** (See Helpful Hints on the next page.)

Helpful Hints and Reminders: Each pregnancy risk category (**A**, **B**, **C**, **D**, or **X**) is explained on the last page of this section.

1. There are no studies of topical exposure to salicylic acid in pregnancy. The risk is probably low since topical salicylic acid is common in many over-the-counter dermatologic agents, and adverse reports are lacking.

Remember: All pregnancies have a background risk of 3% or more for a serious birth defect, even when mom doesn't take a drug of any kind. If you are pregnant or planning a pregnancy, always let your healthcare provider know before taking any drug, prescription or non-prescription, or herbal remedy.

Equate® Anti-Itch Hydrocortisone 1% Cream

Active Ingredient:	Pregnancy Risk Category:
Hydrocortisone 1%	Hydrocortisone has two pregnancy risk categories: **C** when used in the second or third trimesters of pregnancy; **D** if used in the first trimester. (See Helpful Hints below.)

Helpful Hints and Reminders: Each pregnancy risk category (**A**, **B**, **C**, **D**, or **X**) is explained on the last page of this section.

1. Topical corticosteroids should be used in pregnancy only if the potential benefit for mom outweighs the potential risk to her fetus. This class of drug should not be used extensively in pregnant women, in large amounts or for extensive periods of time, especially during the first trimester.

Remember: All pregnancies have a background risk of 3% or more for a serious birth defect, even when mom doesn't take a drug of any kind. If you are pregnant or planning a pregnancy, always let your healthcare provider know before taking any drug, prescription or non-prescription, or herbal remedy.

Equate® Extra Strength Anti-Itch Cream

Active Ingredient:	Pregnancy Risk Category:
Diphenhydramine Hcl	B
Zinc acetate	A

Helpful Hints and Reminders: Each pregnancy risk category (**A**, **B**, **C**, **D**, or **X**) is explained on the last page of this section.

Remember: All pregnancies have a background risk of 3% or more for a serious birth defect, even when mom doesn't take a drug of any kind. If you are pregnant or planning a pregnancy, always let your healthcare provider know before taking any drug, prescription or non-prescription, or herbal remedy.

Equate® Maximum Strength Vagicaine Anti-Itch Cream

Active Ingredient:	Pregnancy Risk Category:
Benzocaine	C
Resorcinol	**Risk is undetermined**, but probably small. The FDA has not assigned a pregnancy risk category to this drug.

Helpful Hints and Reminders: Each pregnancy risk category (**A**, **B**, **C**, **D**, or **X**) is explained on the last page of this section.

Remember: All pregnancies have a background risk of 3% or more for a serious birth defect, even when mom doesn't take a drug of any kind. If you are pregnant or planning a pregnancy, always let your healthcare provider know before taking any drug, prescription or non-prescription, or herbal remedy.

Gold Bond® Maximum Strength Foot Spray, Triple Action Relief

Active Ingredient:	Pregnancy Risk Category:
Menthol 1%	**Risk is undetermined.** (See Helpful Hints below.)

Helpful Hints and Reminders: Each pregnancy risk category (**A**, **B**, **C**, **D**, or **X**) is explained on the last page of this section.

1. There are no studies using menthol in pregnant animals or pregnant women. However, the risk of fetal birth defects is believed to be quite small, according to the Illinois Teratogen Information Service (ITIS).

Remember: All pregnancies have a background risk of 3% or more for a serious birth defect, even when mom doesn't take a drug of any kind. If you are pregnant or planning a pregnancy, always let your healthcare provider know before taking any drug, prescription or non-prescription, or herbal remedy.

Nupercainal® Hemorrhoidal & Topical Analgesic Ointment

Active Ingredient:	Pregnancy Risk Category:
Dubucaine	**C**

Helpful Hints and Reminders: Each pregnancy risk category (**A**, **B**, **C**, **D**, or **X**) is explained on the last page of this section.

Remember: All pregnancies have a background risk of 3% or more for a serious birth defect, even when mom doesn't take a drug of any kind. If you are pregnant or planning a pregnancy, always let your healthcare provider know before taking any drug, prescription or non-prescription, or herbal remedy.

Preparation H® Cooling Gel

Active Ingredient:	Pregnancy Risk Category:
Phenylephrine Hcl	C
Witch hazel	**Fetal risk is undetermined**. (See Helpful Hints below.)

Helpful Hints and Reminders: Each pregnancy risk category (**A**, **B**, **C**, **D**, or **X**) is explained on the last page of this section.

1. The FDA has not assigned a pregnancy risk category to witch hazel. Fetal risk may be quite small since evidence of fetal harm has not been reported and very little of this ingredient is absorbed into mom's circulation.

Remember: All pregnancies have a background risk of 3% or more for a serious birth defect, even when mom doesn't take a drug of any kind. If you are pregnant or planning a pregnancy, always let your healthcare provider know before taking any drug, prescription or non-prescription, or herbal remedy.

Preparation H® Cream

Active Ingredient:	Pregnancy Risk Category:
Glycerine	C
Phenylephrine Hcl	C
Pramoxine Hcl	C
White petrolatum	**Risk is undetermined**. (See Helpful Hints below.)

Helpful Hints and Reminders: Each pregnancy risk category (**A**, **B**, **C**, **D**, or **X**) is explained on the last page of this section.

1. The FDA has not assigned a pregnancy risk category to white petrolatum. Fetal risk may be quite small since evidence of fetal harm has not been reported and very little of this ingredient is absorbed into mom's circulation.

Remember: All pregnancies have a background risk of 3% or more for a serious birth defect, even when mom doesn't take a drug of any kind. If you are pregnant or planning a pregnancy, always let your healthcare provider know before taking any drug, prescription or non-prescription, or herbal remedy.

Preparation H® Hydrocortisone 1%

Active Ingredient:	Pregnancy Risk Category:
Hydrocortisone 1%	Hydrocortisone has two pregnancy risk categories: **C** when used in the second or third trimesters of pregnancy; **D** if used in the first trimester.

Helpful Hints and Reminders: Each pregnancy risk category (**A**, **B**, **C**, **D**, or **X**) is explained on the last page of this section.

1. Topical corticosteroids should be used in pregnancy only if the potential benefit for mom outweighs the potential risk to her fetus. This class of drug should not be used extensively in pregnant women, in large amounts or for extensive periods of time, especially during the first trimester.

Remember: All pregnancies have a background risk of 3% or more for a serious birth defect, even when mom doesn't take a drug of any kind. If you are pregnant or planning a pregnancy, always let your healthcare provider know before taking any drug, prescription or non-prescription, or herbal remedy.

Preparation H® Ointment

Active Ingredient:	Pregnancy Risk Category:
Phenylephrine Hcl	C
Mineral Oil	C

(continued)

Shark liver oil	**Risk is undetermined**. (See Helpful Hints below.)
Petrolatum	**Risk is undetermined**. (See Helpful Hints below.)

Helpful Hints and Reminders: Each pregnancy risk category (**A**, **B**, **C**, **D**, or **X**) is explained on the last page of this section.

1. The FDA has not assigned a pregnancy risk category to shark liver oil or petrolatum. Fetal risk may be quite small since evidence of fetal harm has not been reported and very little of these ingredients are absorbed into mom's circulation.

Remember: All pregnancies have a background risk of 3% or more for a serious birth defect, even when mom doesn't take a drug of any kind. If you are pregnant or planning a pregnancy, always let your healthcare provider know before taking any drug, prescription or non-prescription, or herbal remedy.

Preparation H® Suppositories

Active Ingredient:	Pregnancy Risk Category:
Phenylephrine Hcl	C
Cocoa butter	**Risk is undetermined**. (See Helpful Hints below.)
Shark liver oil	**Risk is undetermined**. (See Helpful Hints below.)

Helpful Hints and Reminders: Each pregnancy risk category (**A**, **B**, **C**, **D**, or **X**) is explained on the last page of this section.

1. The FDA has not assigned a pregnancy risk category to cocoa butter or shark liver oil. Fetal risk may be quite small since evidence of fetal harm has not been reported and very little of these ingredients are absorbed into mom's circulation.

Remember: All pregnancies have a background risk of 3% or more for a serious birth defect, even when mom doesn't take a drug of any kind.

If you are pregnant or planning a pregnancy, always let your healthcare provider know before taking any drug, prescription or non-prescription, or herbal remedy.

Solarcaine® Aloe Extra Burn Relief Spray

Active Ingredient:	Pregnancy Risk Category:
Lidocaine Hcl	B

Helpful Hints and Reminders: Each pregnancy risk category (**A**, **B**, **C**, **D**, or **X**) is explained on the last page of this section.

Remember: All pregnancies have a background risk of 3% or more for a serious birth defect, even when mom doesn't take a drug of any kind. If you are pregnant or planning a pregnancy, always let your healthcare provider know before taking any drug, prescription or non-prescription, or herbal remedy.

Solarcaine® Cool Aloe Burn Relief Formula Pain Relieving Gel With Lidocaine Hcl

Active Ingredient:	Pregnancy Risk Category:
Lidocaine Hcl	B

Helpful Hints and Reminders: Each pregnancy risk category (**A**, **B**, **C**, **D**, or **X**) is explained on the last page of this section.

Remember: All pregnancies have a background risk of 3% or more for a serious birth defect, even when mom doesn't take a drug of any kind. If you are pregnant or planning a pregnancy, always let your healthcare provider know before taking any drug, prescription or non-prescription, or herbal remedy.

Tucks® Hemorrhoidal Ointment

Solarcaine® First Aid Medicated Spray

Active Ingredient:	Pregnancy Risk Category:
Benzocaine	C
Triclosan	**Risk is undetermined**. The FDA has not assigned a pregnancy risk category to this drug.

Helpful Hints and Reminders: Each pregnancy risk category (**A**, **B**, **C**, **D**, or **X**) is explained on the last page of this section.

Remember: All pregnancies have a background risk of 3% or more for a serious birth defect, even when mom doesn't take a drug of any kind. If you are pregnant or planning a pregnancy, always let your healthcare provider know before taking any drug, prescription or non-prescription, or herbal remedy.

Tronolane® Anesthetic Hemorrhoid Cream

Active Ingredient:	Pregnancy Risk Category:
Pramoxine	C
Zinc oxide	C

Helpful Hints and Reminders: Each pregnancy risk category (**A**, **B**, **C**, **D**, or **X**) is explained on the last page of this section.

Remember: All pregnancies have a background risk of 3% or more for a serious birth defect, even when mom doesn't take a drug of any kind. If you are pregnant or planning a pregnancy, always let your healthcare provider know before taking any drug, prescription or non-prescription, or herbal remedy.

Tucks® Hemorrhoidal Ointment

Active Ingredient:	Pregnancy Risk Category:
Mineral oil	C
Pramoxine Hcl	C
Zinc oxide	C

Helpful Hints and Reminders: Each pregnancy risk category (**A**, **B**, **C**, **D**, or **X**) is explained on the last page of this section.

Remember: All pregnancies have a background risk of 3% or more for a serious birth defect, even when mom doesn't take a drug of any kind. If you are pregnant or planning a pregnancy, always let your healthcare provider know before taking any drug, prescription or non-prescription, or herbal remedy.

Tucks® Hydrocortisone Anti-Itch Ointment

Active Ingredient:	Pregnancy Risk Category:
Hydrocortisone acetate	Hydrocortisone has two pregnancy risk categories: **C** when used in the second or third trimesters of pregnancy; **D** if used in the first trimester.

Helpful Hints and Reminders: Each pregnancy risk category (**A**, **B**, **C**, **D**, or **X**) is explained on the last page of this section.

1. Topical corticosteroids should be used in pregnancy only if the potential benefit for mom outweighs the potential risk to her fetus. This class of drug should not be used extensively in pregnant women, in large amounts or for extensive periods of time, especially during the first trimester.

Remember: All pregnancies have a background risk of 3% or more for a serious birth defect, even when mom doesn't take a drug of any kind. If you are pregnant or planning a pregnancy, always let your healthcare provider know before taking any drug, prescription or non-prescription, or herbal remedy.

Up & Up™ Analgesic Cream Rub

Active Ingredient:	Pregnancy Risk Category:
Trolamine salicylate	**Risk is undetermined.** The FDA has not assigned a pregnancy risk category to this active ingredient. However, there have been no reports of fetal harm using this drug, and a relatively small amount of this drug is absorbed into mom's bloodstream, meaning very little, if any, reaches the fetus.

Helpful Hints and Reminders: Each pregnancy risk category (**A**, **B**, **C**, **D**, or **X**) is explained on the last page of this section.

Remember: All pregnancies have a background risk of 3% or more for a serious birth defect, even when mom doesn't take a drug of any kind. If you are pregnant or planning a pregnancy, always let your healthcare provider know before taking any drug, prescription or non-prescription, or herbal remedy.

Up & Up™ Epsom Salts

Active Ingredient:	Pregnancy Risk Category:
Magnesium sulfate	B

Helpful Hints and Reminders: Each pregnancy risk category (**A**, **B**, **C**, **D**, or **X**) is explained on the last page of this section.

Remember: All pregnancies have a background risk of 3% or more for a serious birth defect, even when mom doesn't take a drug of any kind. If you are pregnant or planning a pregnancy, always let your healthcare provider know before taking any drug, prescription or non-prescription, or herbal remedy.

The FDA's Pregnancy Risk Categories: A, B, C, D, X

Adapted to the Active Ingredients in Nonprescription drugs

Category A: Controlled studies using the active ingredient in pregnant women have not shown harmful fetal effects throughout pregnancy, and the possibility of fetal harm seems remote. My comment: *Though apparently safe, these active ingredients should still only be used in pregnancy when clearly indicated.*

Category B: Either studies have shown no evidence of fetal harm when using the active ingredient in pregnant animals, but no controlled studies have been done in pregnant women, **or** studies have shown evidence of fetal harm when using the active ingredient in pregnant animals, but controlled studies in pregnant women have not shown evidence of fetal harm. My comment: *These active ingredients should only be used in pregnancy when clearly indicated.*

Category C: Either studies have shown evidence of fetal harm when using the active ingredient in pregnant animals, but no controlled studies have been done in pregnant women, **or** studies using the active ingredient in pregnant animals have not been done, and studies of pregnant women are insufficient to reach a conclusion. These active ingredients should only be used by a pregnant woman if the potential benefit justifies the potential risk of fetal harm, which, in many cases, is unknown. My comment: *It's impossible to calculate the potential risk of fetal harm when, in many cases, it's unknown. Thus, these active ingredients should only be used in pregnancy when clearly needed.*

Category D: Studies have shown evidence of fetal harm when using the active ingredient in pregnant women. However, the potential benefit of using the active ingredient in some life-threatening situations for

mom may outweigh the potential risk of fetal harm. For example, when mom requires cancer treatment or when she has a serious disease for which safer active ingredients cannot be used or are less effective. My comment: *These exceptional indications rarely occur when considering a nonprescription drug in pregnancy.*

Category X: My comment: *Because the risk of fetal harm is too high, no Category X active ingredients have been approved for use in nonprescription drugs.*

Active Ingredients Assigned Two Pregnancy Risk Categories: Some active ingredients have two pregnancy risk categories, depending on which trimester of pregnancy the active ingredient is used. For example, naproxen sodium, the active ingredient in Aleve, belongs to Category **B** when used in the first and second trimesters of pregnancy. If used in the third trimester, however, the active ingredient belongs to Category **D**. My comment: *This means naproxen sodium should not be used in the third trimester unless prescribed by a physician who has advised her patient of the risks involved.*

Section 12: Sleep Aids

Advil® PM Caplets & Liqui-Gels®

Active Ingredient:	Pregnancy Risk Category:
Diphenhydramine	B
Ibuprofen	Ibuprofen has two pregnancy risk categories: **B** when used in the first or second trimesters of pregnancy; **D** if used in the third trimester. (See Helpful Hints below.)

Helpful Hints and Reminders: Each pregnancy risk category (**A**, **B**, **C**, **D**, or **X**) is explained on the last page of this section.

1. Ibuprofen is a member of the non-steroidal, anti-inflammatory family of drugs, or NSAIDs. Members of this family of drugs should not be used during the third trimester of pregnancy (last 12 weeks) unless specifically prescribed by a clinician. See the Appendix for "Non-Steroidal, Anti-Inflammatory Drugs (NSAIDs) in Pregnancy," which describes the serious problems these drugs may cause for unborn babies when taken in the third trimester of pregnancy.

2. Women attempting to conceive should not use any NSAID, including Ibuprofen, because of the findings in animals that

these drugs may block implantation of the early embryo in the wall of the uterus, in effect preventing pregnancy.

Remember: All pregnancies have a background risk of 3% or more for a serious birth defect, even when mom doesn't take a drug of any kind. If you are pregnant or planning a pregnancy, always let your healthcare provider know before taking any drug, prescription or non-prescription, or herbal remedy.

Compoz® Nighttime Sleep Aid

Active Ingredient:	Pregnancy Risk Category:
Diphenhydramine Hcl	B

Helpful Hints and Reminders: Each pregnancy risk category (**A**, **B**, **C**, **D**, or **X**) is explained on the last page of this section.

Remember: All pregnancies have a background risk of 3% or more for a serious birth defect, even when mom doesn't take a drug of any kind. If you are pregnant or planning a pregnancy, always let your healthcare provider know before taking any drug, prescription or non-prescription, or herbal remedy.

CVS® Maximum Strength Nighttime Sleep Aid 50 mg Softgels

Active Ingredient:	Pregnancy Risk Category:
Diphenhydramine Hcl	B

Helpful Hints and Reminders: Each pregnancy risk category (**A**, **B**, **C**, **D**, or **X**) is explained on the last page of this section.

Remember: All pregnancies have a background risk of 3% or more for a serious birth defect, even when mom doesn't take a drug of any kind. If you are pregnant or planning a pregnancy, always let your healthcare provider know before taking any drug, prescription or non-prescription, or herbal remedy.

CVS® Nighttime Sleep Aid Caplets

Active Ingredient:	Pregnancy Risk Category:
Diphenhydramine Hcl	B

Helpful Hints and Reminders: Each pregnancy risk category (**A**, **B**, **C**, **D**, or **X**) is explained on the last page of this section.

Remember: All pregnancies have a background risk of 3% or more for a serious birth defect, even when mom doesn't take a drug of any kind. If you are pregnant or planning a pregnancy, always let your healthcare provider know before taking any drug, prescription or non-prescription, or herbal remedy.

CVS® Nighttime Sleep-Aid Tablets

Active Ingredient:	Pregnancy Risk Category:
Doxylamine succinate	A

Helpful Hints and Reminders: Each pregnancy risk category (**A**, **B**, **C**, **D**, or **X**) is explained on the last page of this section.

Remember: All pregnancies have a background risk of 3% or more for a serious birth defect, even when mom doesn't take a drug of any kind. If you are pregnant or planning a pregnancy, always let your healthcare provider know before taking any drug, prescription or non-prescription, or herbal remedy.

CVS® Sleep Aid Mini-Caplets Nighttime

Active Ingredient:	Pregnancy Risk Category:
Diphenhydramine Hcl	B

Helpful Hints and Reminders: Each pregnancy risk category (**A**, **B**, **C**, **D**, or **X**) is explained on the last page of this section.

Remember: All pregnancies have a background risk of 3% or more for a serious birth defect, even when mom doesn't take a drug of any kind. If you are pregnant or planning a pregnancy, always let your healthcare

provider know before taking any drug, prescription or non-prescription, or herbal remedy.

Equate® Ibuprofen PM Caplets Pain Reliever/Sleep Aid

Active Ingredient:	Pregnancy Risk Category:
Diphenhydramine citrate	**B**
Ibuprofen	Ibuprofen has two pregnancy risk categories: **B** when used in the first or second trimesters of pregnancy; **D** if used in the third trimester. (See Helpful Hints below.)

Helpful Hints and Reminders: Each pregnancy risk category (**A**, **B**, **C**, **D**, or **X**) is explained on the last page of this section.

1. Ibuprofen is a member of the non-steroidal, anti-inflammatory family of drugs, or NSAIDs. Members of this family of drugs should not be used during the third trimester of pregnancy (last 12 weeks) unless specifically prescribed by a clinician. See the Appendix for "Non-Steroidal, Anti-Inflammatory Drugs (NSAIDs) in Pregnancy," which describes the serious problems these drugs may cause for unborn babies when taken in the third trimester of pregnancy.

2. Women attempting to conceive should not use any NSAID, including Ibuprofen, because of the findings in animals that these drugs may block implantation of the early embryo in the wall of the uterus, in effect preventing pregnancy.

Remember: All pregnancies have a background risk of 3% or more for a serious birth defect, even when mom doesn't take a drug of any kind. If you are pregnant or planning a pregnancy, always let your healthcare provider know before taking any drug, prescription or non-prescription, or herbal remedy.

Equate® Nighttime Mini-Caplets Sleep Aid

Active Ingredient:	Pregnancy Risk Category:
Doxylamine	A

Helpful Hints and Reminders: Each pregnancy risk category (**A**, **B**, **C**, **D**, or **X**) is explained on the last page of this section.

Remember: All pregnancies have a background risk of 3% or more for a serious birth defect, even when mom doesn't take a drug of any kind. If you are pregnant or planning a pregnancy, always let your healthcare provider know before taking any drug, prescription or non-prescription, or herbal remedy.

Equate® Sleep Aid Tablets

Active Ingredient:	Pregnancy Risk Category:
Doxylamine	A

Helpful Hints and Reminders: Each pregnancy risk category (**A**, **B**, **C**, **D**, or **X**) is explained on the last page of this section.

Remember: All pregnancies have a background risk of 3% or more for a serious birth defect, even when mom doesn't take a drug of any kind. If you are pregnant or planning a pregnancy, always let your healthcare provider know before taking any drug, prescription or non-prescription, or herbal remedy.

Kirkland Signature™ Sleep Aid, Doxylamine Succinate Tablets

Active Ingredient:	Pregnancy Risk Category:
Doxylamine succinate	A

Helpful Hints and Reminders: Each pregnancy risk category (**A**, **B**, **C**, **D**, or **X**) is explained on the last page of this section.

Remember: All pregnancies have a background risk of 3% or more for a serious birth defect, even when mom doesn't take a drug of any kind.

If you are pregnant or planning a pregnancy, always let your healthcare provider know before taking any drug, prescription or non-prescription, or herbal remedy.

Rite Aid® Nighttime Sleep Aid Mini Caplets

Active Ingredient:	Pregnancy Risk Category:
Diphenhydramine Hcl	B

Helpful Hints and Reminders: Each pregnancy risk category (**A**, **B**, **C**, **D**, or **X**) is explained on the last page of this section.

Remember: All pregnancies have a background risk of 3% or more for a serious birth defect, even when mom doesn't take a drug of any kind. If you are pregnant or planning a pregnancy, always let your healthcare provider know before taking any drug, prescription or non-prescription, or herbal remedy.

Sominex® Maximum Strength Formula

Active Ingredient:	Pregnancy Risk Category:
Diphenhydramine	B

Helpful Hints and Reminders: Each pregnancy risk category (**A**, **B**, **C**, **D**, or **X**) is explained on the last page of this section.

Remember: All pregnancies have a background risk of 3% or more for a serious birth defect, even when mom doesn't take a drug of any kind. If you are pregnant or planning a pregnancy, always let your healthcare provider know before taking any drug, prescription or non-prescription, or herbal remedy.

Sominex® Original Formula

Active Ingredient:	Pregnancy Risk Category:
Diphenhydramine	B

Helpful Hints and Reminders: Each pregnancy risk category (**A**, **B**, **C**, **D**, or **X**) is explained on the last page of this section.

Remember: All pregnancies have a background risk of 3% or more for a serious birth defect, even when mom doesn't take a drug of any kind. If you are pregnant or planning a pregnancy, always let your healthcare provider know before taking any drug, prescription or non-prescription, or herbal remedy.

Tylenol® PM Simply Sleep

Active Ingredient:	Pregnancy Risk Category:
Diphenhydramine Hcl	B

Helpful Hints and Reminders: Each pregnancy risk category (**A**, **B**, **C**, **D**, or **X**) is explained on the last page of this section.

Remember: All pregnancies have a background risk of 3% or more for a serious birth defect, even when mom doesn't take a drug of any kind. If you are pregnant or planning a pregnancy, always let your healthcare provider know before taking any drug, prescription or non-prescription, or herbal remedy.

Unisom® PM Pain SleepCaps

Active Ingredient:	Pregnancy Risk Category:
Diphenhydramine Hcl	B
Acetaminophen	B

Helpful Hints and Reminders: Each pregnancy risk category (**A**, **B**, **C**, **D**, or **X**) is explained on the last page of this section.

Remember: All pregnancies have a background risk of 3% or more for a serious birth defect, even when mom doesn't take a drug of any kind. If you are pregnant or planning a pregnancy, always let your healthcare provider know before taking any drug, prescription or non-prescription, or herbal remedy.

Unisom® SleepTabs

Unisom® SleepGels

Active Ingredient:	Pregnancy Risk Category:
Diphenhydramine Hcl	B

Helpful Hints and Reminders: Each pregnancy risk category (**A**, **B**, **C**, **D**, or **X**) is explained on the last page of this section.

Remember: All pregnancies have a background risk of 3% or more for a serious birth defect, even when mom doesn't take a drug of any kind. If you are pregnant or planning a pregnancy, always let your healthcare provider know before taking any drug, prescription or non-prescription, or herbal remedy.

Unisom® SleepMelts

Active Ingredient:	Pregnancy Risk Category:
Diphenhydramine Hcl	B

Helpful Hints and Reminders: Each pregnancy risk category (**A**, **B**, **C**, **D**, or **X**) is explained on the last page of this section.

Remember: All pregnancies have a background risk of 3% or more for a serious birth defect, even when mom doesn't take a drug of any kind. If you are pregnant or planning a pregnancy, always let your healthcare provider know before taking any drug, prescription or non-prescription, or herbal remedy.

Unisom® SleepTabs

Active Ingredient:	Pregnancy Risk Category:
Doxylamine succinate	A

Helpful Hints and Reminders: Each pregnancy risk category (**A**, **B**, **C**, **D**, or **X**) is explained on the last page of this section.

Remember: All pregnancies have a background risk of 3% or more for a serious birth defect, even when mom doesn't take a drug of any kind. If you are pregnant or planning a pregnancy, always let your healthcare

provider know before taking any drug, prescription or non-prescription, or herbal remedy.

Up & Up™ Maximum Strength Sleep Aid

Active Ingredient:	Pregnancy Risk Category:
Diphenhydramine Hcl	B

Helpful Hints and Reminders: Each pregnancy risk category (**A**, **B**, **C**, **D**, or **X**) is explained on the last page of this section.

Remember: All pregnancies have a background risk of 3% or more for a serious birth defect, even when mom doesn't take a drug of any kind. If you are pregnant or planning a pregnancy, always let your healthcare provider know before taking any drug, prescription or non-prescription, or herbal remedy.

The FDA's Pregnancy Risk Categories: A, B, C, D, X

Adapted to the Active Ingredients in Nonprescription drugs

Category A: Controlled studies using the active ingredient in pregnant women have not shown harmful fetal effects throughout pregnancy, and the possibility of fetal harm seems remote. My comment: *Though apparently safe, these active ingredients should still only be used in pregnancy when clearly indicated.*

Category B: Either studies have shown no evidence of fetal harm when using the active ingredient in pregnant animals, but no controlled studies have been done in pregnant women, **or** studies have shown evidence of fetal harm when using the active ingredient in pregnant animals, but controlled studies in pregnant women have not shown evidence of fetal harm. My comment: *These active ingredients should only be used in pregnancy when clearly indicated.*

Category C: Either studies have shown evidence of fetal harm when using the active ingredient in pregnant animals, but no controlled studies have been done in pregnant women, **or** studies using the active ingredient in pregnant animals have not been done, and studies of pregnant women are insufficient to reach a conclusion. These active ingredients should only be used by a pregnant woman if the potential benefit justifies the potential risk of fetal harm, which, in many cases, is unknown. My comment: *It's impossible to calculate the potential risk of fetal harm when, in many cases, it's unknown. Thus, these active ingredients should only be used in pregnancy when clearly needed.*

Category D: Studies have shown evidence of fetal harm when using the active ingredient in pregnant women. However, the potential benefit of using the active ingredient in some life-threatening situations for

mom may outweigh the potential risk of fetal harm. For example, when mom requires cancer treatment or when she has a serious disease for which safer active ingredients cannot be used or are less effective. My comment: *These exceptional indications rarely occur when considering a nonprescription drug in pregnancy.*

Category X: My comment: *Because the risk of fetal harm is too high, no Category X active ingredients have been approved for use in nonprescription drugs.*

Active Ingredients Assigned Two Pregnancy Risk Categories: Some active ingredients have two pregnancy risk categories, depending on which trimester of pregnancy the active ingredient is used. For example, naproxen sodium, the active ingredient in Aleve, belongs to Category **B** when used in the first and second trimesters of pregnancy. If used in the third trimester, however, the active ingredient belongs to Category **D**. My comment: *This means naproxen sodium should not be used in the third trimester unless prescribed by a physician who has advised her patient of the risks involved.*

Section 13: Smoking Cessation Aids

Equate® Stop Smoking Aid Nicotine Lozenge 2 Mg Mint or Cherry

Active Ingredient:	Pregnancy Risk Category:
Nicotine Polacrilex	**D** (See Helpful Hint below.)

Helpful Hints and Reminders: Each pregnancy risk category (**A**, **B**, **C**, **D**, or **X**) is explained on the last page of this section.

1. If you become pregnant while taking any form of nicotine replacement therapy, contact your healthcare provider immediately for advice.

Remember: All pregnancies have a background risk of 3% or more for a serious birth defect, even when mom doesn't take a drug of any kind. If you are pregnant or planning a pregnancy, always let your healthcare provider know before taking any drug, prescription or non-prescription, or herbal remedy.

Equate® Stop Smoking Aid Nicotine Original Flavor Gum 4 Mg

Active Ingredient:	Pregnancy Risk Category:
Nicotine Polacrilex	**D** (See Helpful Hint below.)

Helpful Hints and Reminders: Each pregnancy risk category (**A**, **B**, **C**, **D**, or **X**) is explained on the last page of this section.

1. If you become pregnant while taking any form of nicotine replacement therapy, contact your healthcare provider immediately for advice.

Remember: All pregnancies have a background risk of 3% or more for a serious birth defect, even when mom doesn't take a drug of any kind. If you are pregnant or planning a pregnancy, always let your healthcare provider know before taking any drug, prescription or non-prescription, or herbal remedy.

Up & Up™ Nicotine 2 mg & 4 mg Polacrilex Gum

Active Ingredient:	Pregnancy Risk Category:
Nicotine	**D** (See Helpful Hint below.)

Helpful Hints and Reminders: Each pregnancy risk category (**A**, **B**, **C**, **D**, or **X**) is explained on the last page of this section.

1. If you become pregnant while taking any form of nicotine replacement therapy, contact your healthcare provider immediately for advice.

Remember: All pregnancies have a background risk of 3% or more for a serious birth defect, even when mom doesn't take a drug of any kind. If you are pregnant or planning a pregnancy, always let your healthcare provider know before taking any drug, prescription or non-prescription, or herbal remedy.

Up & Up™ Nicotine Patches

Active Ingredient:	Pregnancy Risk Category:
Nicotine	**D** (See Helpful Hint below.)

Helpful Hints and Reminders: Each pregnancy risk category (**A**, **B**, **C**, **D**, or **X**) is explained on the last page of this section.

1. If you become pregnant while taking any form of nicotine replacement therapy, contact your healthcare provider immediately for advice.

Remember: All pregnancies have a background risk of 3% or more for a serious birth defect, even when mom doesn't take a drug of any kind. If you are pregnant or planning a pregnancy, always let your healthcare provider know before taking any drug, prescription or non-prescription, or herbal remedy.

The FDA's Pregnancy Risk Categories: A, B, C, D, X

Adapted to the Active Ingredients in Nonprescription drugs

Category A: Controlled studies using the active ingredient in pregnant women have not shown harmful fetal effects throughout pregnancy, and the possibility of fetal harm seems remote. My comment: *Though apparently safe, these active ingredients should still only be used in pregnancy when clearly indicated.*

Category B: Either studies have shown no evidence of fetal harm when using the active ingredient in pregnant animals, but no controlled studies have been done in pregnant women, **or** studies have shown evidence of fetal harm when using the active ingredient in pregnant animals, but controlled studies in pregnant women have not shown evidence of fetal harm. My comment: *These active ingredients should only be used in pregnancy when clearly indicated.*

Category C: Either studies have shown evidence of fetal harm when using the active ingredient in pregnant animals, but no controlled studies have been done in pregnant women, **or** studies using the active ingredient in pregnant animals have not been done, and studies of pregnant women are insufficient to reach a conclusion. These active ingredients should only be used by a pregnant woman if the potential benefit justifies the potential risk of fetal harm, which, in many cases, is unknown. My comment: *It's impossible to calculate the potential risk of fetal harm when, in many cases, it's unknown. Thus, these active ingredients should only be used in pregnancy when clearly needed.*

Category D: Studies have shown evidence of fetal harm when using the active ingredient in pregnant women. However, the potential benefit of using the active ingredient in some life-threatening situations for

mom may outweigh the potential risk of fetal harm. For example, when mom requires cancer treatment or when she has a serious disease for which safer active ingredients cannot be used or are less effective. My comment: *These exceptional indications rarely occur when considering a nonprescription drug in pregnancy.*

Category X: My comment: *Because the risk of fetal harm is too high, no Category X active ingredients have been approved for use in nonprescription drugs.*

Active Ingredients Assigned Two Pregnancy Risk Categories: Some active ingredients have two pregnancy risk categories, depending on which trimester of pregnancy the active ingredient is used. For example, naproxen sodium, the active ingredient in Aleve, belongs to Category **B** when used in the first and second trimesters of pregnancy. If used in the third trimester, however, the active ingredient belongs to Category **D**. My comment: *This means naproxen sodium should not be used in the third trimester unless prescribed by a physician who has advised her patient of the risks involved.*

Section 14: The Remainder

NoDoz® Maximum Strength

Active Ingredient:	Pregnancy Risk Category:
Caffeine	B

Helpful Hints and Reminders: Each pregnancy risk category (**A**, **B**, **C**, **D**, or **X**) is explained on the last page of this section.

Remember: All pregnancies have a background risk of 3% or more for a serious birth defect, even when mom doesn't take a drug of any kind. If you are pregnant or planning a pregnancy, always let your healthcare provider know before taking any drug, prescription or non-prescription, or herbal remedy.

Target® Lice Treatment Shampoo

Active Ingredient:	Pregnancy Risk Category:
Piperonyl butoxide + Pyrethrum extract	Combination pregnancy risk category – **C**

Helpful Hints and Reminders: Each pregnancy risk category (**A**, **B**, **C**, **D**, or **X**) is explained on the last page of this section.

Remember: All pregnancies have a background risk of 3% or more for a serious birth defect, even when mom doesn't take a drug of any kind.

Vivarin® Caffeine Alertness Aid

If you are pregnant or planning a pregnancy, always let your healthcare provider know before taking any drug, prescription or non-prescription, or herbal remedy.

Vivarin® Caffeine Alertness Aid

Active Ingredient:	Pregnancy Risk Category:
Caffeine	B

Helpful Hints and Reminders: Each pregnancy risk category (**A**, **B**, **C**, **D**, or **X**) is explained on the last page of this section.

Remember: All pregnancies have a background risk of 3% or more for a serious birth defect, even when mom doesn't take a drug of any kind. If you are pregnant or planning a pregnancy, always let your healthcare provider know before taking any drug, prescription or non-prescription, or herbal remedy.

The FDA's Pregnancy Risk Categories: A, B, C, D, X

Adapted to the Active Ingredients in Nonprescription drugs

Category A: Controlled studies using the active ingredient in pregnant women have not shown harmful fetal effects throughout pregnancy, and the possibility of fetal harm seems remote. My comment: *Though apparently safe, these active ingredients should still only be used in pregnancy when clearly indicated.*

Category B: Either studies have shown no evidence of fetal harm when using the active ingredient in pregnant animals, but no controlled studies have been done in pregnant women, **or** studies have shown evidence of fetal harm when using the active ingredient in pregnant animals, but controlled studies in pregnant women have not shown evidence of fetal harm. My comment: *These active ingredients should only be used in pregnancy when clearly indicated.*

Category C: Either studies have shown evidence of fetal harm when using the active ingredient in pregnant animals, but no controlled studies have been done in pregnant women, **or** studies using the active ingredient in pregnant animals have not been done, and studies of pregnant women are insufficient to reach a conclusion. These active ingredients should only be used by a pregnant woman if the potential benefit justifies the potential risk of fetal harm, which, in many cases, is unknown. My comment: *It's impossible to calculate the potential risk of fetal harm when, in many cases, it's unknown. Thus, these active ingredients should only be used in pregnancy when clearly needed.*

Category D: Studies have shown evidence of fetal harm when using the active ingredient in pregnant women. However, the potential benefit of using the active ingredient in some life-threatening situations for

mom may outweigh the potential risk of fetal harm. For example, when mom requires cancer treatment or when she has a serious disease for which safer active ingredients cannot be used or are less effective. My comment: *These exceptional indications rarely occur when considering a nonprescription drug in pregnancy.*

Category X: My comment: *Because the risk of fetal harm is too high, no Category X active ingredients have been approved for use in nonprescription drugs.*

Active Ingredients Assigned Two Pregnancy Risk Categories: Some active ingredients have two pregnancy risk categories, depending on which trimester of pregnancy the active ingredient is used. For example, naproxen sodium, the active ingredient in Aleve, belongs to Category **B** when used in the first and second trimesters of pregnancy. If used in the third trimester, however, the active ingredient belongs to Category **D**. My comment: *This means naproxen sodium should not be used in the third trimester unless prescribed by a physician who has advised her patient of the risks involved.*

A Three-Step Process for Creating a Pregnancy Risk Profile of the Active Ingredients in a Nonprescription Drug©

Three-Step Process:

The first step in creating your own pregnancy risk profile for the active ingredients in a nonprescription drug is to **identify the drug's active ingredients**. Nonprescription drugs typically have from one to five active ingredients that treat the patient's symptoms and are actually drugs themselves. Since all nonprescription drug labels now have the same format, you will always find the active ingredients listed on the first line of the drug label or "Drug Facts." For example, under "Drug Facts" on a bottle of Tylenol, acetaminophen is listed on the first line as the only active ingredient.

Having identified the drug's active ingredients (In Tylenol's case there is only one – acetaminophen), **the second step** is to **find the pregnancy risk category (A, B, C, D, X) for each active ingredient** in the "Table of Active Ingredients and Their Pregnancy Risk Categories" shown on page 298. Continuing with the Tylenol example, when you look up acetaminophen in the Table, you find that the pregnancy risk category for acetaminophen is **B**. Now, **for the third step**, all you need is the **explanation for pregnancy risk category B**, which is found after the Table.

To Summarize: Using Tylenol as an example, we have now created a pregnancy risk profile of the active ingredients in a nonprescription drug using the three-step process: **First**, we read the first line of "Drug Facts" and discovered that Tylenol has one active ingredient, which is acetaminophen. **Second**, we looked up acetaminophen in our "Table of Active Ingredients and Their Pregnancy Risk Categories" and discovered that acetaminophen has a pregnancy risk category of **B**. **Third**, we read the explanation for pregnancy risk category **B** at the end of the Table and decided a **B** rating means Tylenol is probably safe to take throughout pregnancy. However, acetaminophen, like all other category **B** active ingredients, should only be used in pregnancy when clearly indicated.

Some active ingredients like aspirin, ibuprofen, and naproxen sodium have two pregnancy risk categories, depending on which trimester of pregnancy the drug is used. These three drugs are members of the non-steroidal, anti-inflammatory family of drugs, or NSAIDs. Since they may seriously harm the fetus if used in the third trimester, they have been assigned to pregnancy risk category **D** if used during the last 12 weeks of pregnancy. (For more details, see "Non-Steroidal, Anti-Inflammatory Drugs in Pregnancy," in the Appendix.)

Now, here's another example of how you might use our "Table of Active Ingredients and Their Pregnancy Risk Categories". Let's say you have a Kindle or an iPad and have downloaded this book to your digital device. You have just hung up the phone after making an appointment with your OB's office. The call for an appointment was prompted by a positive home pregnancy test result just this morning.

Giddy with excitement, you calm down long enough to make up a list of over-the-counter drugs you are taking. You want to know if the active ingredients in those drugs are safe for unborn babies. First, you write down folic acid. This is one of many active ingredients in a multivitamin you've been taking daily ever since you and your husband started planning your pregnancy. Next, you list ibuprofen, the active ingredient in generic ibuprofen, which you take frequently for the pain of arthritis. Finally, you've been taking Zantac for heartburn, but it's not in the book. However, the drug label says the only active ingredient is ranitidine, which reduces stomach acid.

Next, you scroll through the "Table of Active Ingredients and Their Pregnancy Risk Categories" and find that the pregnancy risk category for folic acid is **A**. You repeat the process for ibuprofen and find its pregnancy risk category is **B** when used in the first or second trimesters of pregnancy; **D** if used in the third trimester. You also discover that the pregnancy risk category for ranitidine is **B**.

The following day you keep your appointment with your OB and go over what you have learned. You both agree that it's safe to continue taking your folic acid and the Zantac, because the pregnancy risk categories for their active ingredients are **A** and **B** respectively. But your doctor suggests that you stop taking ibuprofen and switch to acetaminophen. You scroll down your list of active ingredients and note that acetaminophen is category **B**.

Your doctor asks if he can see your iPad. He is so impressed with the "Three Step Approach to Finding the Pregnancy Risk Categories for the Active Ingredients in Nonprescription Drugs" that he decides to buy an iPad and digitally download this book for the office. "We get asked questions about over-the-counter drugs in pregnancy all the time," he said. "Now I can answer with facts and not have to say, over and over, 'I don't know.' "

Table of Active Ingredients and Their Pregnancy Risk Category

Active Ingredient:	Pregnancy Risk Category:
Acetaminophen	B
Aluminum hydroxide	C
Aspirin	Aspirin has two pregnancy risk categories: **C** when used in the first or second trimesters of pregnancy; **D** if used in the third trimester. See the appendix for "Non-Steroidal, Anti-inflammatory Drugs (NSAIDs) in Pregnancy" for further details.
Bacitracin	C
Benzocaine	C

(continued)

Benzoyl peroxide	C
Bisacodyl	C
Bismuth subsalicylate	Although the pregnancy risk category for this drug is C, some experts believe this drug should only be taken during the first half of pregnancy since significant adverse fetal effects have occasionally occurred from chronic exposure to salicylates.
Brompheniramine maleate	C
Butenafine hydrochloride	C
Butoconazole nitrate	C
Caffeine	B
Calcium carbonate	C
Calcium polycarbophil	C
Camphor	C
Cascara	C
Castor Oil	C
Cetirizine hydrochloride	B
Chlorcyclizine	C
Chlorpheniramine maleate	B
Cimetidine	B
Clemastine fumarate	B
Clotrimazole	B
Cromolyn sodium	B
Cyclizine hydrochloride	B
Danthron	C
Desloradine	C
Dexbrompheniramine maleate	C
Dexchlorpheniramine maleate	B
Dextromethorphan	C

(continued)

Dibucaine	C
Dimenhydrinate	B
Diphenhydramine hydrochloride	B
Diphenhydramine monocitrate	B
Docosanol	B
Docusate sodium	C
Doxylamine succinate	A
Dyclonine hydrochloride	C
Ephedrine sulfate	C
Epinephrine hydrochloride	C
Famotidine	B
Folic acid	A
Garlic	C
Ginger	C
Ginseng	C
Glycerin	C
Guaifenesin	C
Haloprogin	B
Hydrocortisone	C when used in the second or third trimesters of pregnancy; D if used in the first trimester.
Ibuprofen	Ibuprofen has two pregnancy risk categories: B when used in the first or second trimesters of pregnancy; D if used in the third trimester. See the appendix for "Non-Steroidal, Anti-inflammatory Drugs (NSAIDs) in Pregnancy" for further details.
Iodine	D
Kaolin	C
Ketoconazole	C

(*continued*)

Ketoprofen	Ketoprofen has two pregnancy risk categories: **B** when used in the first or second trimesters of pregnancy; **D** if used in the third trimester. See the appendix for Non-Steroidal, Anti-inflammatory Drugs (NSAIDs) in Pregnancy" for further details.
Ketotifen	C
Lansoprazole	B
Lidocaine	B
Loperamide	B
Loratadine	B
Magnesium hydroxide	C
Magnesium sulfate	B
Meclizine	B
Methylcellulose	C
Miconazole nitrate	C
Mineral oil	C
Minoxidil	C
Naphazoline	C
Naproxen sodium	Naproxen sodium has two pregnancy risk categories: **C** when used in the first or second trimesters of pregnancy; **D** if used in the third trimester. See the appendix for Non-Steroidal, Anti-inflammatory Drugs (NSAIDs) in Pregnancy" for further details.
Neomycin	C
Nicotine (Gum, lozenges, nasal spray, skin patches)	D
Nizatidine	B
Omeprazole	C
Orlistat	B

Oxymetazoline hydrochloride	C
Paregoric	B
Peppermint	C
Permethrin	B
Pheniramine maleate	C
Phenylephrine hydrochloride	C
Phenylpropanolamine hydrochloride	C
Podophyllin	C
Polycarbophil	C
Polyethylene glycol 3350	C
Polymyxin B	B
Povidone-iodine	D
Pramoxine	C
Pseudoephedrine hydrochloride	C
Pseudoephedrine sulfate	C
Psyllium	B
Pyrethrin + Piperonyl Butoxide	C for the combination
Pyrantel pamoate	C
Pyrilamine	C
Ranitidine	B
Senna	C
Simethicone	C
Sodium Bicarbonate	C
Terbinafine hydrochloride	B
Tetracaine	C
Tioconazole	C
Tolnaftate	C
Triprolidine hydrochloride	C
Xylometazoline hydrochloride	C
Zinc Acetate	A
Zinc Oxide	C

The FDA's Pregnancy Risk Categories: A, B, C, D, X

Adapted to the Active Ingredients in Nonprescription drugs

Category A: Controlled studies using the active ingredient in pregnant women have not shown harmful fetal effects throughout pregnancy, and the possibility of fetal harm seems remote. My comment: *Though apparently safe, these active ingredients should still only be used in pregnancy when clearly indicated.*

Category B: Either studies have shown no evidence of fetal harm when using the active ingredient in pregnant animals, but no controlled studies have been done in pregnant women, **or** studies have shown evidence of fetal harm when using the active ingredient in pregnant animals, but controlled studies in pregnant women have not shown evidence of fetal harm. My comment: *These active ingredients should only be used in pregnancy when clearly indicated.*

Category C: Either studies have shown evidence of fetal harm when using the active ingredient in pregnant animals, but no controlled studies have been done in pregnant women, **or** studies using the active ingredient in pregnant animals have not been done, and studies of pregnant women are insufficient to reach a conclusion. These active ingredients should only be used by a pregnant woman if the potential benefit justifies the potential risk of fetal harm, which, in many cases, is unknown. My comment: *It's impossible to calculate the potential risk of fetal harm when, in many cases, it's unknown. Thus, these active ingredients should only be used in pregnancy when clearly needed.*

Category D: Studies have shown evidence of fetal harm when using the active ingredient in pregnant women. However, the potential benefit of using the active ingredient in some life-threatening situations for

mom may outweigh the potential risk of fetal harm. For example, when mom requires cancer treatment or when she has a serious disease for which safer active ingredients cannot be used or are less effective. My comment: *These exceptional indications rarely occur when considering a nonprescription drug in pregnancy.*

Category X: My comment: *Because the risk of fetal harm is too high, no Category X active ingredients have been approved for use in nonprescription drugs.*

Active Ingredients Assigned Two Pregnancy Risk Categories: Some active ingredients have two pregnancy risk categories, depending on which trimester of pregnancy the active ingredient is used. For example, naproxen sodium, the active ingredient in Aleve, belongs to Category **B** when used in the first and second trimesters of pregnancy. If used in the third trimester, however, the active ingredient belongs to Category **D**. My comment: *This means naproxen sodium should not be used in the third trimester unless prescribed by a physician who has advised her patient of the risks involved.*

Appendix - 1

NON-STEROIDAL, ANTI-INFLAMMATORY DRUGS (NSAIDS) IN PREGNANCY

The non-steroidal, anti-inflammatory drugs are commonly used to reduce the inflammation and pain associated with arthritis, rheumatoid arthritis, and osteoarthritis.[8] Of the 21 different NSAIDs on the market, including aspirin, only four have been approved for over-the-counter use as active ingredients in nonprescription drugs. These four are aspirin, ibuprofen, ketoprofen, and naproxen sodium.

In the past, members of this family of drugs have been associated with the following complications (usually described in case reports) when used in the third trimester of pregnancy:

- Persistent pulmonary hypertension in the fetus, meaning high blood pressure in the lungs. This potentially life-threatening condition causes breathing problems at birth, the need for intensive care, and has led to death.
- Decreased fetal kidney function, leading to a lack of amniotic fluid since fetal urine is the main source of amniotic fluid; crowding in the womb and compression of the fetal chest, leading to failure of fetal lungs to fully develop before birth; and life-threatening breathing problems at birth.
- After birth, infection and perforation of the newborn intestine, leading to peritonitis and the need for emergency surgery in the newborn period.
- Bleeding in the newborn brain.

These potential effects apply to all NSAIDs, whether purchased by prescription or over-the-counter. As a result, all NSAIDs have been assigned a pregnancy risk category of **D** if used in the third trimester of pregnancy. This means a pregnant woman should not take one of these drugs alone or in combination with other active ingredients during the third trimester except under the rare circumstance when a prescribing physician believes potential benefit for mom, who has a serious health problem, outweighs potential fetal risk.

In general, acetaminophen is the over-the-counter pain reliever and fever reducer of choice in pregnancy. However, it has a dark side too. For more, turn the page and read "Taking Acetaminophen: The Good and The Ugly."

Appendix - 2

TAKING ACETAMINOPHEN: THE GOOD AND THE UGLY

Acetaminophen, the active ingredient in Tylenol, is probably the most popular drug for treating fever and pain in the United States.

- Acetaminophen is found in more than 90 prescription drugs and over-the-counter products, including narcotic pain relievers and cough-and-cold remedies.
- Acetaminophen is generally considered safe and is the recommended pain and fever reliever in pregnancy. But, if you take too much and overdose, it can be toxic to your liver. Herein lies the problem, especially if you are pregnant and two lives are at stake.
- Acetaminophen is the leading cause of acute liver failure in the United States. In some cases, the overdose is intentional while in others, the overdose is unintentional.
- **Intentional cases** of acetaminophen-related acute liver failure are due to attempted suicide, amounting to roughly half the cases.
- **Unintentional cases** are usually due to unintentional overdosing. Why? Because patients didn't realize they were taking more than one drug containing acetaminophen.
- In 2006 alone, the American Association of Poison Control Centers implicated acetaminophen in nearly 140,000 poisoning cases (an average of 383 cases per day, nationwide), in which more than 100 patients died. The drug is responsible for more emergency room visits than any other drug on the market.

- Acetaminophen's toxic effect on the liver is directly related to the amount of acetaminophen consumed daily. Experts have set the maximum safe daily dose of acetaminophen at 4,000 mg per day. The directions on a bottle of Tylenol Arthritis caplets say to take two caplets every eight hours, not to exceed six caplets per day. Each caplet contains 650 mg of acetaminophen. Thus the total daily recommended dose is six times 650 mg or 3,900 mg, which is 100 mg less than the maximum safe daily dose of 4,000 mg.

- Obviously, if you are taking another medication that also contains acetaminophen, you will easily exceed the maximum safe daily dose, increasing your risk of liver damage and acute liver failure. The following case example illustrates this point.

Case Example: You are 36 weeks pregnant and broke your arm yesterday when you fell on the ice. Fortunately, your unborn baby did not suffer any ill effects from the fall. After the doctor placed your arm in a cast, she prescribed Vicodin, two tablets every six hours, for pain. Unknown to you, Vicodin contains 5 mg of hydrocodone and 500 mg of acetaminophen per tablet. As instructed, you are taking two tablets every six hours for a total of 8 tablets per day. This equals 4,000 mg of acetaminophen daily (eight tablets × 500 mg/tablet equals 4,000 mg), the maximum safe daily dose.

You come down with a cough, stuffy nose, chills, a fever, and ache all over. So you drag yourself to the corner drugstore and buy a bottle of Sudafed PE, Severe Cold pills, which contain three active ingredients: a decongestant for your stuffy nose, a cough suppressant for your cough, and acetaminophen for your fever and aching. Each pill contains 325 mg of acetaminophen. The directions say to take two pills every four hours, up to a maximum of 12 pills per day. If you follow those directions, you will be taking 12 × 325 mg of acetaminophen per pill for 3,900 mg daily. Adding this amount to the 4,000 mg of acetaminophen you are already taking for your broken arm, the total daily dose of acetaminophen will be 7,900 mg, almost double the safe daily dose of 4,000 mg.

The message? Never take more than one drug at a time that contains acetaminophen, pregnant or not. If unsure, read the labels carefully, ask the pharmacist when you purchase the medicines, or call your doctor.

Source: Cleveland Clinic Journal of Medicine. Vol. 77, No. 1, pages 19-27, Jan. 2010

Partial List of Prescription & Non-Prescription Drugs Containing Acetaminophen

Prescription Drugs:

Narcotics: Darvocet-N 50 & 100 Tablets; Esgic Tablets or Capsules; Esgic-Plus Tablets; Fioricet Tablets; Fioricet With Codeine Capsules; Hycomine Compound Tablets; Hydrocet Capsules; Lorcet-HD Capsules; Lorcet 10/650 Tablets; Loratab 2.5/500 Tablets; Loratab 5/500 Tablets; Loratab 7.5/500 Tablets; Loratab 10/500 Tablets; Lortab Elixir; Midrin Capsules; Norco Tablets; Percocet Tablets; Phenaphen with Codeine No. 3 Capsules; Phrenilin Forte Capsules & Tablets; Roxicet Tablets, Caplets, and Oral Solution; Sedapap Tablets 60/650; Talacen Caplets; Tylenol with Codeine #2, #3, & #4 Tablets; Tylenol with Codeine Elixir; Tylox Capsules; Vicodin Tablets; Vicodin ES Tablets; Vicodin HP Tablets; Wygesic Tablets; Zydone Capsules; Zydone Tablets.

Non-Prescription Drugs:

Cold & Flu Medications: Alka-Seltzer Plus Cold and Cough family of medicines; Benadryl Allergy/Cold Tablets; Children's Cepacol Sore

Throat Formula Liquids; Comtrex Deep Chest Cold & Congestion Relief Liquigels; Comtrex Maximum-Strength Multi-Symptom Acute Head Cold & Sinus Pressure Relief Tablets; Contac Severe Cold & Flu Caplets Maximum Strength; Coricidin D Decongestant Tablets; Coricidin HBP Cold & Flu Tablets; Coricidin HBP Nighttime Cold & Cough Liquid; Dimetapp Cold and Fever Suspension; Drixoral Cold & Flu Extended-Release Tablets; Robitussin Cold, Cough & Flu Liqui-Gel medicines; Sudafed Severe Cold & Cough medicines, Theraflu Maximum Strength Nighttime Flu, Cold, & Cough Hot Liquid & Caplets; Theraflu Flu, Cold, and Cough medicines; Triaminic Severe Cold & Fever medicines; Triaminicin Tablets; Children's Tylenol Cold and Flu medicines; Infants' Tylenol Cold medicines; Tylenol Cold medications/ Tylenol Flu medications; Tylenol Flu Nighttime Maximum Strength Gelcaps; Vicks 44M Cough, Cold & Flu Relief; Vicks DayQuil medicines, Vicks NyQuil medicines.

Pain Relievers: Aspirin Free Excedrin Geltabs and Caplets; Excedrin Extra-Strength Tablets, Geltabs, and Caplets; Excedrin Migraine Caplets and Tablets; Tylenol Extra Strength Adult Liquid Pain Reliever; Tylenol Arthritis Extended Relief Caplets; Tylenol Extra Strength Gelcaps, Geltabs, Caplets and Tablets; Infants' Tylenol Concentrated Drops; Tylenol Regular Strength Caplets and Tablets.

Sleep Aids: Excedrin PM Caplets, Geltabs, and Tablets; Tylenol PM Extra Strength Pain Reliever/Sleep Aid Caplets, Geltabs, and Gelcaps; Unisom with Pain Relief.

Menstrual Pain: Lurline PMS Tablets; Maximum Strength Midol Menstrual; Maximum Strength Midol PMS; Maximum Strength Midol Teen; Teen Midol Caplets.

Allergy/Sinus: Benadryl Allergy/Sinus medicines; Drixoral Allergy/ Sinus Extended-Release Tablets; Sine-Aid Maximum Strength Sinus medications; Sinulin Tablets; Sinutab Sinus Allergy medications; Sudafed Sinus Caplets & Tablets; Tavist Sinus Caplets and Gelcaps; Tylenol Allergy Sinus Maximum Strength medications; Children's Tylenol Sinus medicines; Children's Tylenol Sinus Medicines; Tylenol Severe Allergy medication; Tylenol Sinus, Maximum Strength Geltabs, Gelcaps, Caplets, and Tablets.[9]

Appendix - 3

REFERENCES

1. Consumer Healthcare Products Association. FAQs About the Regulation of OTCs. www.chpa-info.org

2. Consumer Healthcare Products Association. FAQs About Rx-to-OTC Switch. www.chpa-info.org

3. Consumer Healthcare Products Association. Ingredients & Dosages Transferred from Rx-to-OTC Status (or New OTC Approvals) by the Food and Drug Administration Since 1975. September 23, 2010. www.chpa-info.org

4. CHPA Educational Foundation. Check the OTC Label. www.OTCsafety.org

5. Federal Register 1980: 37434–67.

6. Federal Register 2008; Volume 73, No. 104: 30831 – 30868.

7. Schilling, A and Colleagues. Acetaminophen: Old Drug, New Warnings. Cleveland Clinic Journal of Medicine. Vol. 77 (1): 19 – 27, Jan. 2010.

8. Briggs, G.C., Nonsteroidal anti-inflammatory drugs. OB/GYN News. Jan. 1, 2004.

9. Things to Consider When Prescribing Medications That Contain Acetaminophen. Knoll Pharmaceutical Company, Mount Olive, NJ, 2000.

10. United States Patent & Trademark Office and Company Web Sites. September 23, 2010.

* * * *

Sources for Random Sample of 500 Nonprescription Drugs & Their Active Ingredients

- PDR for Nonprescription Drugs, Dietary Supplements, and Herbs (28, 29, 30 edition; 2008, 2009, 2010 respectively) Thomson Healthcare Inc, Montvale, NJ 07645-1725.
- CHPA's Pocket Primer on OTC Active Ingredients, Online Update, April 2010. Consumer Healthcare Products Association, Washington, DC, 20006.
- Approved Drug Products with Therapeutic Equivalence Evaluations, 30th Edition. U.S. Department of Health and Human Services. 2010.
- The drug products themselves.

Appendix - 4

TRADEMARKS FOR THE OVER-THE-COUNTER DRUGS IN THIS BOOK[10]

4-Way® is a registered trademark of Novartis AG.

Abreva® is a registered trademark of Smithkline Beecham Corporation.

Actifed® is a registered trademark of Warner-Lambert Company.

Advil® is a registered trademark of Wyeth LLC.

Afrin® is a registered trademark of Schering Corporation.

Alavert® is a registered trademark of Wyeth LLC.

Aleve® is a registered trademark of Bayer Healthcare LLC

Alka-Seltzer® is a registered trademark of Bayer Healthcare LLC.

Allerest® is a registered trademark of Insight Pharmaceuticals LLC.

Alophen® is a registered trademark of Numark laboratories.

Anacin® is a registered trademark of Insight Pharmaceuticals LLC.

Ascriptin® is a registered trademark of Novartis AG.

Aveeno® is a registered trademark of Johnson & Johnson Corporation.

Axid® is a registered trademark of GlaxoSmithKline LLC.

Bayer® is a registered trademark of Bayer AG.

Benadryl Allergy Plus® is a registered trademark of Johnson & Johnson LLC.

Benadryl-D® is a registered trademark of Johnson & Johnson LLC.

Benylin® is a registered trademark of Warner-Lambert.

Bonine® is a registered trademark of Insight Pharmaceuticals LLC.

Buckley's® is a registered trademark of Buckley's Limited Corporation.

Bufferin® is a registered trademark of Novartis AG.

Carter's Little Pills® is a registered trademark of Church & Dwight Corporation.

Chlor-Trimeton® is a registered trademark of Schering Corporation.

Claritin® is a registered trademark of Schering Corporation.

Colace® is a registered trademark of Purdue Products LP.

Compoz® is a registered trademark of Medtech Laboratories Inc.

Comtrex® is a registered trademark of Novartis AG.

Contac® is a registered trademark of GlaxoSmithKline.

Coricidin® HBP is a registered trademark of Schering Corporation.

Correctol® is a registered trademark of Schering-Plough Healthcare Products.

Cortaid® is a registered trademark of Johnson & Johnson Corporation.

CVS® is a registered trademark of CVS Pharmacy Corporation.

DayQuil® is a registered trademark of Procter & Gamble Company.

Delsym® is a registered trademark of Reckitt Benckiser Corporation.

Dermarest® is a registered trademark of Church & Dwight Company.

Desenex® is a registered trademark of Novartis AG.

Diabetic Tussin® is a registered trademark of Hi-Tech Pharmacal Company.

Dimetapp® is a registered trademark of Wyeth LLC.

Dramamine® is a registered trademark of Johnson & Johnson Corporation.

Dristan® is a registered trademark of Wyeth LLC.

Appendix - 4

Dulcolax® is a registered trademark of Boehringer Ingelheim Pharmaceuticals.

Equate® is a registered trademark of Wal-Mart Stores Inc.

Excedrin® is a registered trademark of Novartis AG.

Ex-Lax® is a registered trademark of Novartis AG.

Fibercon® is a registered trademark of Wyeth holdings Corporation.

Gas-X® is a registered trademark of Novartis AG.

Gaviscon® is a registered trademark of GlaxoSmithKline.

Gelusil® is a registered trademark of Wellspring Pharmaceutical Corporation.

Gold Bond® is a registered trademark of Sanofin Aventis.

Goody's® is a registered trademark of GlaxoSmithKline.

Imodium® is a registered trademark of Johnson & Johnson Corporation.

Kirkland Signature™ is a registered trademark of Costco Wholesale Corporation.

Lamisil AT® is a registered trademark of Novartis AG.

Maalox® is a registered trademark of Novartis AG.

Marezine® is a registered trademark of Himmel Pharmaceuticals Corporation.

Metamucil® is a registered trademark of Procter & Gamble Company.

Midol® is a registered trademark of Bayer Healthcare LLC.

Miralax® is a registered trademark of Schering-Plough Healthcare Products.

Motrin 1B® is a registered trademark of Johnson & Johnson Corporation.

Mucinex® is a registered trademark of Reckitt Benckiser Corporation.

Mylanta® is a registered trademark of Johnson & Johnson-Merck Partnership.

NasalCrom® is a registered trademark of Blacksmith Brands Inc.

Neosporin® is a registered trademark of Johnson & Johnson Corporation.

NoDoz® is a registered trademark of Novartis AG.

Nupercainal® is a registered trademark of Novartis AG.

NyQuil® is a registered trademark of Procter & Gamble Company.

Pepcid® AC® is a registered trademark of Johnson & Johnson-Merck Partnership.

Pepto-Bismol® is a registered trademark of Procter & Gamble Company.

Peri-Colace® is a registered trademark of Purdue Products LP.

Phillips® is a registered trademark of Bayer Healthcare LLC.

Polysporin® is a registered trademark of Monarch Pharmaceuticals Corporation.

Preparation H® is a registered trademark of Wyeth LLC.

Prilosec OTC® is a registered trademark of Astra Zeneca.

Primatene® is a registered trademark of Wyeth LLC.

Rite Aid® is a registered trademark of Name Rite LLC.

Robitussin® is a registered trademark of Wyeth LLC.

Rolaids® is a registered trademark of Warner-Lambert Company.

Rugby® is a registered trademark of Rugby Laboratories Inc.

St. Joseph® is a registered trademark of McNeil PPC.

Solarcaine® is a registered trademark of Schering-Plough Healthcare Products.

Sominex® is a registered trademark of GlaxoSmithKline LLC.

Sudafed® is a registered trademark of Johnson & Johnson Corporation.

Sudafed OM® is a registered trademark of Johnson & Johnson Corporation.

Sudafed PE® is a registered trademark of Warner-Lambert Company.

Target® is a registered trademark of Target Brands Inc.

Tavist D® is a registered trademark of Novartis AG.

Theraflu® is a registered trademark of Novartis AG.

Triptone® is a registered trademark of Church & Dwight Company.

Tronolane® is a registered trademark of Abbott Laboratories.

Tucks® is a registered trademark of Warner-Lambert Company.

Tums® Smoothies is a registered trademark of GlaxoSmithKline LLC.

Tylenol® is a registered trademark of Tylenol Company.

Tylenol® PM is a registered trademark of Tylenol Company.

Unisom® is a registered trademark of Sanofi Aventis.

Up & Up™ is a registered trademark of Target Brands Inc.

Vagistat-1® is a registered trademark of Novartis AG.

Vicks® Formula 44® is a registered trademark of Procter & Gamble Company.

Vivarin® is a registered trademark of GlaxoSmithKline LLC.

Walgreens® is a registered trademark of Walgreen Company.

XL-3® is a registered trademark of Marvi Asesores.

Zantac® is a registered trademark of Johnson & Johnson Corporation.

Zegerid OTC™ Capsules is a registered trademark of Schering-Plough Healthcare Products.

Zicam® is a registered trademark of Zicam LLC.

Zyrtec-D® is a registered trademark of UCB Pharma SA.

Source: United States Patent & Trademark Office and Company Web Sites. September 23, 2010

Index of 500 Over-The-Counter-Drugs in This Book

OTC Drug Name	Section(s)
4-Way® Fast Acting Nasal Spray: Nasal Decongestant	2
4-Way® Menthol: Nasal Decongestant	2
4-Way® Moisturing Relief Nasal Decongestant	2
Abreva® Pump & Original Tube	5
Actifed® Cold & Allergy Tablets	1, 2
Advil® Allergy Sinus Caplets	1
Advil® Cold & Sinus Caplets & Liqui-Gels®	2
Advil® Migraine Capsules	10
Advil® Multi-Symptom Cold Caplets	2
Advil® PM Caplets & Liqui-Gels®	10, 12
Advil® Tablets, Caplets, Gel Caplets & Liqui-Gel® Caplets	10
Afrin® 12 Hour Spray, Sinus	1, 2
Afrin® All Night No Drip, Nasal Spray	1, 2
Afrin® No Drip 12 Hour Pump Mist, Extra Moisturizing	1, 2
Afrin® No Drip 12 Hour Pump Mist, Severe Congestion	1, 2

(continued)

Index of 500 Over-The-Counter-Drugs in This Book **319**

OTC Drug Name	Section(s)
Afrin® No Drip Original 12 Hour Pump Mist	1, 2
Alavert® Allergy & Sinus D-12 Hour Tablets	1
Alavert® Tablets	1
Aleve® All Day Strong Pain Reliever, Fever Reducer, Caplets	10
Alka-Seltzer Plus® Cherry Burst Cold Formula	2
Alka-Seltzer Plus® Cold & Cough Formula Liquid Gels	2
Alka-Seltzer Plus® Cold & Cough Formula Tablets	2
Alka-Seltzer Plus® Day & Night Cold Formula Liquid Gels	2
Alka-Seltzer Plus® Day & Night Cold Formula Tablets	2
Alka-Seltzer Plus® Day Non-Drowsy Cold Formula	2
Alka-Seltzer Plus® Fast Crystal Packs	2
Alka-Seltzer Plus® Flu Formula	2
Alka-Seltzer Plus® Mucus & Congestion – Liquid Gels	2
Alka-Seltzer Plus® Night Cold Formula	2
Alka-Seltzer Plus® Night Cold Formula Liquid Gels	2
Alka-Seltzer Plus® Orange Zest Cold Formula	2
Alka-Seltzer Plus® Sparkling Original Cold Formula	2
Allerest® PE Allergy & Sinus Relief Tablets	1
Alophen® Tablets	3
Anacin® Extra Strength Aspirin Free	10
Anacin® Max Strength Tablets	10
Anacin® Regular Strength Tablets & Caplets	10
Ascriptin Maximum Strength Pain Reliever Caplets	10
Ascriptin® Tablets Regular Strength	10
Aveeno® Maximum Strength Anti-Itch Cream, 1% Hydrocortisone	11
Axid AR Acid Reducer Tablets	7

(*continued*)

OTC Drug Name	Section(s)
Bayer® AM Extra Strength Aspirin & Alertness Aid Tablets	10
Bayer® Aspirin Extra Strength	10
Bayer® Aspirin Tablets	10
Bayer® Chewable Aspirin, Orange and Cherry	10
Bayer® Extra Strength Back & Body Pain	10
Bayer® Extra Strength Plus	10
Bayer® PM	10
Bayer® Quick Release Crystals	10
Bayer® Women's Low Dose Aspirin	10
Benadryl Extra Strength Itch Relief Stick	11
Benadryl Extra Strength Itch Stopping Cream	11
Benadryl Extra Strength Spray	11
Benadryl Original Strength Itch Stopping Cream	11
Benadryl Readymist Itch Stopping Spray	11
Benadryl® Allergy Kapgels	1
Benadryl® Allergy Quick Dissolve Strips	1
Benadryl® Allergy Ultratab™ Tablets	1
Benadryl® Dye-Free Allergy Liqui-Gels	1
Benadryl-D® Allergy Plus Sinus	1
Benylin® All-in-One® Cold and Flu Caplets	2
Benylin® All-in-One® Cold and Flu Night Caplets	2
Benylin® All-in-One® Cold and Flu Syrup	2
Benylin® All-in-One® Extra Strength Cold & Flu Nighttime Syrup	2
Benylin® Cold & Flu with Codeine	2
Benylin® Cold & Sinus Day/Night Caplets	2
Benylin® Cold & Sinus Plus Caplets	2
Benylin® DM® Tickly Throat & Cough	2
Benylin® DM-D-E® Cough & Chest Congestion with Warming Sensation	2

(continued)

Index of 500 Over-The-Counter-Drugs in This Book

OTC Drug Name	Section(s)
Benylin® DM-D-E® Extra Strength Chest Cough and Cold	2
Benylin® DM-D-E-A® Cough & Cold with Warming Sensation	2
Benylin® DM-E® Extra Strength Chest Cough & Cold	2
Benylin® E® Extra Strength Chest Congestion	2
Benylin® E® Menthol Mucous & Phlegm Relief	2
Benylin® Extra Strength Mucous & Phlegm Relief Plus Cough Control	2
Bonine® Motion Sickness Protection, Raspberry Chewable Tablets	9
Buckley's® Chest Congestion Mixture	2
Buckley's® Cough Mixture	2
Bufferin® Regular and Extra Strength Tablets	10
Carter's® Laxative Tablets	3
Chlor-Trimeton® Allergy Relief, 12 Hour Tablets	1
Chlor-Trimeton® Allergy Relief, 4 Hour Tablets	1
Claritin® 12 Hour Non-Drowsy Reditabs®	1
Claritin® 24 Hour Non-Drowsy Liqui-Gels	1
Claritin® 24 Hour Non-Drowsy Reditabs®	1
Claritin® Eye Itch Relief	1
Claritin® Non-Drowsy Tablets	1
Claritin-D® 12 Hour & 24 Hour Non-Drowsy Tablets	1
Colace® Stool Softener Syrup	3
Colace® Glycerin Suppositories	3
Colace® Stool Softener Capsules	3
Colace® Stool Softener Liquid 1% Solution	3
Compoz® Nighttime Sleep Aid	12
Comtrex® Maximum Strength Day/Night Cold & Cough Caplets	2
Comtrex® Maximum Strength Non-Drowsy Cold & Cough	2

(continued)

OTC Drug Name	Section(s)
Contac® Cold + Flu Day & Night Dual Formula Pack Caplets	2
Contac® Cold + Flu Maximum Strength Caplets	2
Contac® Cold + Flu Non-Drowsy Maximum Strength Caplets	2
Coricidin® HBP Chest Congestion & Cough	2
Coricidin® HBP Cold & Flu	2
Coricidin® HBP Cough & Cold	2
Coricidin® HBP Day & Night Multi-Symptom Cold	2
Coricidin® HBP Maximum Strength Flu	2
Coricidin® HPB Nighttime Multi-Symptom Cold	2
Correctol® Laxative Tablets	3
Cortaid® Advanced 12 Hour Anti-Itch Cream	11
Cortaid® Intensive Therapy Cooling Spray	11
Cortaid® Intensive Therapy Moisturizing Cream	11
Cortaid® Maximum Strength Cream	11
Cortaid® Maximum Strength Ointment	11
CVS® Antacid Liquid Regular Strength Original	7
CVS® Anti-Diarrheal Caplets	4
CVS® Arthritis Pain Relief Caplets Easy Open Bottle	10
CVS® Aspirin 325 Mg Coated Tablets Regular Strength	10
CVS® Aspirin Free Pain Relief PM	10
CVS® Chest Congestion Relief PE Tablets	2
CVS® Cold & Flu BP Tablets	2
CVS® Extra Strength Non-Aspirin PM Caplets	10
CVS® Extra Strength Pain Relief PM Geltabs	10
CVS® Extra Strength Pain Relief PM Rapid Release Gelcaps	10
CVS® Flu & Severe Cold Nighttime Cherry Flavor	2
CVS® Gentle Laxative Suppositories	3

(*continued*)

Index of 500 Over-The-Counter-Drugs in This Book

OTC Drug Name	Section(s)
CVS® Gentle Laxative Tablets	3
CVS® Headache Relief Coated Tablets Added Strength	10
CVS® Ibuprofen PM Pain Reliever Coated Caplets 200 Mg	10
CVS® Maximum Strength Nighttime Sleep Aid 50 mg Softgels	12
CVS® Menstrual Relief, Menstrual Complete Gelcaps or Caplets	8
CVS® Migraine Relief Caplets	10
CVS® Motion Sickness II Tablets Less Drowsy Formula	9
CVS® Motion Sickness Relief Raspberry Flavored Tablet	9
CVS® Motion Sickness Tablets Original Formula	9
CVS® Nighttime Cough & Severe Cold Packets Honey Lemon	2
CVS® Nighttime Sleep Aid Caplets	12
CVS® Nighttime Sleep-Aid Tablets	12
CVS® Pain Relief PM & Pain Relief Caplets Extra Strength	10
CVS® Severe Cold Relief PE Multi-Symptom Caplets	2
CVS® Sinus Congestion & Pain Caplets Daytime & Nighttime	1
CVS® Sleep Aid Mini-Caplets Nighttime	12
CVS® Stomach Relief Caplets	4, 7
CVS® Stomach Relief Liquid Maximum Strength	4
CVS® Stool Softener Capsules Original	3
CVS® Stool Softener Softgels	3
CVS® Tussin Cough Formula Maximum Strength	2
CVS® Tussin DM Cough Suppressant	2
DayQuil® Cold & Flu Relief LiquiCaps	2

(*continued*)

OTC Drug Name	Section(s)
DayQuil® Cold & Flu Relief Liquid	2
DayQuil® Cold & Flu Symptom Relief Plus Vitamin C	2
DayQuil® Cough	2
DayQuil® Mucus Control DM	2
DayQuil® Mucus Control Liquid	2
DayQuil® Sinus LiquiCaps	1
Delsym® Liquid, Grape and Orange Flavors	2
Dermarest® Eczema Medicated Lotion	11
Dermarest® Psoriasis Medicated Skin Treatment	11
Desenex® Antifungal (Shake Powder, Liquid Spray, Spray Powder, Jock Itch Spray & Powder)	5
Desenex® Cream	5
Diabetic Tussin® Cold & Flu Formula	2
Diabetic Tussin® DM Cough Suppressant & Expectorant	2
Diabetic Tussin® DM Maximum Strength Cough Suppressant & Expectorant	2
Diabetic Tussin® EX 400 Expectorant Mucus Relief	2
Diabetic Tussin® EX Expectorant	2
Diabetic Tussin® Night Time Formula Cold, Flu Relief	2
Dimetapp® Cold & Allergy Chewable Tablets	1, 2
Dimetapp® Cold & Allergy Liquid	1, 2
Dimetapp® Cold & Cough	1, 2
Dimetapp® Long Acting Cough Plus Cold	1, 2
Dimetapp® Nighttime Cold & Congestion	1, 2
Dramamine® Chewable Tablets	9
Dramamine® Less Drowsy Formula	9
Dramamine® Original Formula	9
Dristan® Cold Multi-Symptom Nasal Decongestant Coated Tablets	1, 2
Dulcolax® Balance	3

(*continued*)

OTC Drug Name	Section(s)
Dulcolax® Laxative Suppositories	3
Dulcolax® Laxative Tablets	3
Dulcolax® Stool Softener	3
Equate® Clear Lax Polyethylene Glycol 3350 Laxative	3
Equate® 24 Hour Non-Drowsy Allergy Relief, Loratadine Tablets 10 Mg	1
Equate® 75 Mg Acid Reducer	7
Equate® Acetaminophen Extra Strength 500 Mg/ Non-Aspirin/Easy Tabs Pain Reliever	10
Equate® Allergy & Sinus Medication Tablets	1
Equate® Allergy 24 Hour Indoor & Outdoor Tablets	1
Equate® Allergy Medication 25 Mg Antihistamine Capsules	1
Equate® Allergy Relief Liquid	1
Equate® Allergy/Sinus Headache Pain Reliever Caplets	1, 10
Equate® Allergy-D Original Antihistamine/Nasal Decongestant 12 Hour Tablets	1
Equate® Antacid Pink-Bismuth Tablets	4, 7
Equate® Anti-Diarrheal Caplets	4
Equate® Antihistabs Cold & Allergy Relief Tablets	1, 2
Equate® Anti-Itch Hydrocortisone 1% Cream	11
Equate® Arthritis Pain Reliever Caplets	10
Equate® Aspirin Tablets 325 Mg Pain Reliever/Fever Reducer	10
Equate® Chest Congestion Tussin	2
Equate® Chewable Dual Action Acid Reducer Complete Tablets	7
Equate® Cimetidine Tablets, 200 Mg Acid Reducer Heartburn Relief	7
Equate® Cold Head Congestion Severe Pain Reliever Caplets	2

(continued)

OTC Drug Name	Section(s)
Equate® Cold Multi-Symptom Daytime/Nighttime Value Pack Pain Reliever/Fever Reducer 2 pack	2
Equate® Docusate Sodium Stool Softener Softgels	3
Equate® Extra Strength Antacid Tablets	7
Equate® Extra Strength Anti-Itch Cream	11
Equate® Extra Strength Assorted Berries Antacid Tablets	7
Equate® Extra Strength Caplets Pain Reliever/Fever Reducer	10
Equate® Extra Strength Gas Relief Chewable Tablets	6
Equate® Extra Strength Pain Reliever PM Caplets	10
Equate® Ibuprofen 200 Mg Tablets	10
Equate® Ibuprofen PM Caplets Pain Reliever/Sleep Aid	10, 12
Equate® Ibuprofen Softgels 200 Mg Pain Reliever/Fever Reducer	10
Equate® Laxative Fiber Therapy Caplets	3
Equate® Liquid Maximum Strength Original Classic Antacid/Anti-Gas	6, 7
Equate® Loperamide Hydrochloride Tablets 2 Mg Anti-Diarrheal	4
Equate® Maximum Strength Acid Controller & Reducer 20 Mg Tablets	7
Equate® Maximum Strength Laxative Pills	3
Equate® Maximum Strength Vagicaine Anti-Itch Cream	11
Equate® Motion Sickness Tablets	9
Equate® Naproxen Sodium Tablets 220 Mg Pain Reliever/Fever Reducer	10
Equate® Nighttime Mini-Caplets Sleep Aid	12
Equate® Nite Time Cherry Flavor Multi-Symptom Cold/Flu Relief Liquid	2

(*continued*)

OTC Drug Name	Section(s)
Equate® Non-Drowsy Day Time Cold & Flu Multi-Symptom Relief Liquid	2
Equate® Omeprazole Delayed Release Acid Reducer 20 Mg Tablets	7
Equate® Original Effervescent Antacid & Pain Relief	7, 10
Equate® Original Strength Acid Controller Famotidine 10 Mg Tablets	7
Equate® Povidine-Iodine Solution, 10% Topical Microbicide Antiseptic	5
Equate® Regular Strength Liquid Cooling Mint Antacid/Anti-Gas	6, 7
Equate® Severe Allergy & Sinus Headache Maximum Strength Caplets	1
Equate® Sleep Aid Tablets	12
Equate® Stimulant Laxative 5 Mg Tablets	3
Equate® Stop Smoking Aid Nicotine Lozenge 2 Mg Mint or Cherry	13
Equate® Stop Smoking Aid Nicotine Original Flavor Gum 4 Mg	13
Equate® Suphedrine PE Sinus & Allergy Tablets Antihistamine/Nasal Decongestant	1
Equate® Tussin CF Cough & Cold Non-Drowsy	2
Equate® Tussin DM Cough Non-Drowsy Cough Suppressant/Expectorant	2
Equate® Tutti Frutti Flavor Allergy Relief Chewable Tablets	1
Equate® Ultra Strength Tropical Fruit Flavors Antacid Tablets	7
Equate® Women's Bisacodyl Stimulant Laxative Tablets	3
Excedrin® Back and Body Caplets	10
Excedrin® Extra Strength Caplets, Tablets, and Geltabs	10

(*continued*)

OTC Drug Name	Section(s)
Excedrin® Menstrual Complete Express Gels	8
Excedrin® Migraine Pain Reliever Caplets	10
Excedrin® PM Caplets & Tablets	10
Excedrin® Sinus Headache Caplets & Tablets	1
Excedrin® Tension Headache Geltabs, Tablets, and Caplets	10
Ex-Lax® Chocolated Stimulant Laxative	3
Ex-Lax® Laxative Pills, Regular & Maximum Strength	3
Father John's Medicine® Cough Suppressant	2
Fibercon Caplets: Bulk-Forming Laxative	3
Gas-X® Extra Strength: Antigas Softgels & Chewable Tablets	6
Gas-X® Maximum Strength: Antigas Softgels	6
Gas-X® Regular Strength: Antigas Chewable Tablets	6
Gas-X® Thin Strips	6
Gas-X® with Maalox Extra Strength: Chewable Tablets	6
Gaviscon® Extra Strength Chewable Antacid Tablets	7
Gaviscon® Liquid Antacid, Regular Strength, Cool Mint	7
Gelusil® Antacid/Anti-Gas Tablets	6, 7
Gold Bond Maximum Strength Foot Spray, Triple Action Relief	11
Goody's® Body Pain	10
Goody's® Cool Orange	10
Goody's® Extra Strength	10
Goody's® PM	10
Imodium® A-D, Caplets & Mint-Flavored Liquid	4
Imodium® A-D, EZ Chews	4
Imodium® Multi-Symptom Relief, Chewable Tablets & Caplets	4

(*continued*)

Index of 500 Over-The-Counter-Drugs in This Book 329

OTC Drug Name	Section(s)
Kirkland Signature™ Acid Controller Maximum Strength	7
Kirkland Signature™ Acid Reducer Maximum Strength Ranitidine 150 Mg	7
Kirkland Signature™ AllerClear® Non-Drowsy	1
Kirkland Signature™ Allergy Medicine Antihistamine 25 Mg Allergy Relief	1
Kirkland Signature™ Aller-Tec™ Cetirizine HCL Antihistamine	1
Kirkland Signature™ Anti-Diarrheal	4
Kirkland Signature™ Fiber Tabs Bulk-Forming Fiber Laxative	3
Kirkland Signature™ Ibuprofen 200 Mg Tablets	10
Kirkland Signature™ Naproxen Sodium 220 Mg	10
Kirkland Signature™ Omeprazole Acid Reducer 20 mg Delayed Release	7
Kirkland Signature™ Sleep Aid, Doxylamine Succinate Tablets	12
Kirkland Signature™ Suphedrine PE, Nasal & Sinus Decongestant Formula	1
Lamisil AF Defense®: Shake Powder & Spray Powder	5
Lamisil AT® Cream	5
Maalox® Maximum Strength Multi-Symptom Antacid/ Antigas Chewable Tablets	7
Maalox® Maximum Strength Multi-Symptom Antacid/ Antigas Liquid	7
Maalox® Regular Strength Liquid Antacid & Antigas	7
Maalox® Total Stomach Relief	7
Marezine® 50 Mg Motion Sickness Tablets	9
Meclizine HCL, USP 25 Mg, Antiemetic Tablets	9
Metamucil® Fiber Laxative: Powders, Capsules & Wafers	3

(*continued*)

OTC Drug Name	Section(s)
Midol® Complete	8
Midol® Extended Relief	8
Midol® Liquid Gels	8
Midol® PM	8
Midol® Teen Formula	8
MiraLAX® Powder Laxative	3
Motrin® IB Caplets & Tablets	10
Motrin® PM Caplets	10
Mucinex®	2
Mucinex® Cough Mini-Melts™	2
Mucinex® D	2
Mucinex® D Maximum Strength	2
Mucinex® DM	2
Mucinex® DM Maximum Strength	2
Mucinex® Mini-Melts™	2
Mylanta® Gas Maximum Strength Chewable Tablets	6
Mylanta® Gas Maximum Strength Softgels	6
Mylanta® Maximum Strength	7
Mylanta® Regular Strength	7
Mylanta® Supreme	7
Mylanta® Ultimate Strength Chewables	7
Mylanta® Ultimate Strength Liquid	7
NasalCrom® Nasal Allergy Symptom Controller Spray	1
Neosporin® First Aid Antibiotic Ointment	5
Neosporin® First Aid Antiseptic/Pain Relieving Spray	5
Neosporin® Plus Pain Relief, Maximum Strength, First Aid Antibiotic Cream	5
NoDoz® Maximum Strength	14
Nupercainal® Hemorrhoidal & Topical Analgesic Ointment	11

(*continued*)

Index of 500 Over-The-Counter-Drugs in This Book 331

OTC Drug Name	Section(s)
NyQuil® Cold & Flu Relief LiquiCaps	2
NyQuil® Cold & Flu Relief Liquid	2
NyQuil® Cold & Flu Symptom Relief Plus Vitamin C	2
NyQuil® Cough	2
NyQuil® Sinus LiquiCaps	1
Pepcid® AC® Maximum Strength Tablets & EZ Chews	7
Pepcid® AC® Original Strength, Gelcaps & Tablets	7
Pepcid® Complete®, Chewable Tablets Three Flavors	7
Pepto-Bismol®, Original & Maximum Strength	7
Peri-Colace® Tablets	3
Permethrin Lotion 1%	5
Phillips® Genuine Laxative Caplets	3
Phillips® Genuine Milk of Magnesia	3, 7
Polysporin® First Aid Antibiotic Ointment	5
Polysporin® First Aid Antibiotic Powder	5
Preparation H® Cooling Gel	11
Preparation H® Cream	11
Preparation H® Hydrocortisone 1%	11
Preparation H® Ointment	11
Preparation H® Suppositories	11
Prilosec OTC® Tablets	7
Primatene® Mist	1
Rite Aid® Acetaminophen Extended-Release Pain Reliever Tablets	10
Rite Aid® Antacid & Anti-Gas Original	7
Rite Aid® Athlete's Foot Cream Clotrimazole 1% Cream	5
Rite Aid® Extra Strength Gas Relief Softgels	6
Rite Aid® Gas Relief Chewable Tablet Mint Flavor	6

(*continued*)

OTC Drug Name	Section(s)
Rite Aid® Ibuprofen, 200 Mg Coated Tablets	10
Rite Aid® Motion Sickness Relief Tablets	9
Rite Aid® Mucus Relief Chest Immediate-Release Expectorant Tablets	2
Rite Aid® Mucus Relief Sinus Expectorant/ Decongestant	1, 2
Rite Aid® Multi-Symptom Nite Time Cold/Flu Formula	2
Rite Aid® Nighttime Sleep Aid Mini Caplets	12
Rite Aid® Nose Drops	1, 2
Rite Aid® Tussin Cough Suppressant Non-Drowsy	2
Rite Aid® Ultra Strength Gas Relief Softgels	6
Robitussin® Cough & Allergy	1
Robitussin® Cough & Cold CF Liquid	2
Robitussin® Cough & Cold Long Acting	1, 2
Robitussin® Cough & Congestion	2
Robitussin® Cough DM; Robitussin Sugar Free Cough	2
Robitussin® Cough Gels	2
Robitussin® Cough Long Acting	2
Robitussin® Head & Chest Congestion PE	2
Robitussin® Nighttime Cough & Cold	1, 2
Rolaids® Extra Strength Plus Gas Relief Soft Chews (Two flavors)	6, 7
Rolaids® Extra Strength Softchews	7
Rolaids® Extra Strength Tablets (Three flavors)	7
Rolaids® Multi-Symptom Tablets (Two flavors)	6, 7
Rolaids® Regular Strength Tablets (Two flavors)	7
Rugby® Travel Sickness Tablets	9
Solarcaine® Aloe Extra Burn Relief Spray	11
Solarcaine® Cool Aloe Burn Relief Formula Pain Relieving Gel With Lidocaine Hcl	11

(*continued*)

Index of 500 Over-The-Counter-Drugs in This Book

OTC Drug Name	Section(s)
Solarcaine® First Aid Medicated Spray	11
Sominex® Maximum Strength Formula	12
Sominex® Original Formula	12
St. Joseph® 81 Mg Aspirin Enteric Safety-Coated Tablets	10
St. Joseph® 81 Mg Chewable Aspirin	10
Sudafed OM® Sinus Cold Spray	2
Sudafed OM® Sinus Congestion Spray	2
Sudafed PE® Cold and Cough Caplets	2
Sudafed PE® Day & Night Nasal Decongestant Tablets	2
Sudafed PE® Maximum Strength Sinus & Allergy Tablets	1
Sudafed PE® Nasal Decongestant Tablet	1
Sudafed PE® Nighttime Cold Caplets	2
Sudafed PE® Non-Drying Sinus Caplets	1
Sudafed PE® Severe Cold Formula Caplets	2
Sudafed PE® Sinus Headache Caplets	1
Sudafed PE® Triple Action™ Caplets	1
Sudafed® 12 Hour Tablets	1
Sudafed® 24 Hour tablets	1
Sudafed® Nasal Decongestant Tablets	1
Sudafed® Sinus Pain 12 Hour Caplet	1
Sudafed® Triple Action™ Caplets	1
Target® Acetaminophen Pain Relief Caplets	10
Target® Allergy Relief Capsules	1
Target® Antacid Anti-Gas Liquid	7
Target® Antifungal Foot Spray	5
Target® Athlete's Foot Cream	5
Target® Cold PE Daytime Caplets	2

(continued)

Index of 500 Over-The-Counter-Drugs in This Book

OTC Drug Name	Section(s)
Target® Cough Relief DM Liquid	2
Target® Day/Night Cold/Flu Relief Softgels	2
Target® Extra Strength Pain Reliever PM Caplets	10
Target® Famotidine Acid Reducer Complete Mint Chews	7
Target® Famotidine Acid Relief Tablets	7
Target® Lice Treatment Shampoo	14
Target® Maximum Strength Laxative Tablets	3
Target® Maximum Strength Nasal Decongestant PE Tablets	1, 2
Target® Migraine Formula Caplets	10
Target® Multi-Symptom Day/Night Combo Cold Relief Caplets	2
Target® Multi-Symptom Daytime Cold & Flu Softgels	2
Target® Multi-Symptom Nighttime Cold/ Flu Relief Liquid	2
Target® Naproxen Sodium Caplets	10
Target® Nighttime Cold/Flu Relief	2
Target® Omeprazole 20 Mg Acid Relief Tablets	7
Target® Ranitidine Acid Relief Tablets	7
Target® Sinus Congestion & Pain Cool Ice® Caplets	1
Target® Stool Softener & Stimulant Laxative Tablets	3
Target® Stool Softener Soft Gels	3
Target® Sugar-Free Fiber Therapy Laxative Powder	3
Target® Women's Laxative Tablets	3
Tavist® Allergy Tablets	1
Theraflu® Caplets Daytime Severe Cold	2
Theraflu® Caplets Nighttime Severe Cold	2
Theraflu® Cold & Cough	2
Theraflu® Cold & Sore Throat	1, 2
Theraflu® Daytime Severe Cold	2

(continued)

Index of 500 Over-The-Counter-Drugs in This Book **335**

OTC Drug Name	Section(s)
Theraflu® Flu & Chest Congestion	2
Theraflu® Flu & Sore Throat	2
Theraflu® Nighttime Severe Cold	2
Theraflu® Thinstrips Daytime Cold & Cough	2
Theraflu® Thinstrips Nighttime Cold & Cough	2
Theraflu® Warming Relief Daytime Severe Cold	2
Theraflu® Warming Relief Nighttime Severe Cold	2
Triptone® For Motion Sickness Tablets	9
Tronolane® Anesthetic Hemorrhoid Cream	11
Tucks® Hemorrhoidal Ointment	11
Tucks® Hydrocortisone Anti-Itch Ointment	11
Tums® E-X 750 (Four flavors)	7
Tums® E-X Sugar Free	7
Tums® New Dual Action (Two flavors)	7
Tums® New Quik Pak	7
Tums® Regular Strength (Two flavors)	7
Tums® Smoothies (Five flavors)	7
Tums® Ultra 1000 (Four flavors)	7
Tylenol® 8 Hour	10
Tylenol® Allergy Multi-Symptom	1
Tylenol® Allergy Multi-Symptom Nighttime	1
Tylenol® Arthritis Pain	10
Tylenol® Cold Head Congestion Day/Night Pack	2
Tylenol® Cold Head Congestion Daytime	2
Tylenol® Cold Head Congestion Nighttime	2
Tylenol® Cold Head Congestion Severe	2
Tylenol® Cold Multi-Symptom Day/Night Pack	2
Tylenol® Cold Multi-Symptom Daytime	2
Tylenol® Cold Multi-Symptom Nighttime	2
Tylenol® Cold Multi-Symptom Severe	2

(continued)

OTC Drug Name	Section(s)
Tylenol® Cold Severe Congestion Daytime	2
Tylenol® Extra Strength	10
Tylenol® PM	10
Tylenol® PM Simply Sleep	12
Tylenol® Regular Strength	10
Tylenol® Sinus Congestion and Pain Day/Night Pack	1
Tylenol® Sinus Congestion and Pain Daytime	1
Tylenol® Sinus Congestion and Pain Nighttime	1
Tylenol® Sinus Congestion and Pain Severe	1
Unisom® PM Pain SleepCaps	10, 12
Unisom® SleepGels	12
Unisom® SleepMelts	12
Unisom® SleepTabs	12
Up & Up™ Allergy & Cold Relief	1
Up & Up™ Analgesic Cream Rub	11
Up & Up™ Bismuth Stomach Relief	4
Up & Up™ Epsom Salts	11
Up & Up™ Ibuprofen Pain Relief 200 Mg	10
Up & Up™ Maximum Strength Sleep Aid	12
Up & Up™ Mucus Relief DM	2
Up & Up™ Nicotine 2 Mg & 4 Mg Polacrilex Gum	13
Up & Up™ Nicotine Patches	13
Vagistat-1 (Tioconazole Ointment 6.5%	5
Vicks® Formula 44® Custom Care™ Body Aches	10
Vicks® Formula 44® Custom Care™ Chesty Cough	2
Vicks® Formula 44® Custom Care™ Congestion	2
Vicks® Formula 44® Custom Care™ Cough & Cold PM	2
Vicks® Formula 44® Custom Care™ Dry Cough Suppressant	2

(*continued*)

Index of 500 Over-The-Counter-Drugs in This Book 337

OTC Drug Name	Section(s)
Vicks® Formula 44® Custom Care™ Sore Throat Lozenges	10
Vicks® Formula 44® Custom Care™ Sore Throat Spray	10
Vicks® Sinex® VapoSpray™ 12-hour Decongestant Nasal Spray	2
Vicks® Sinex® VapoSpray™ 12-Hour Decongestant UltraFine Mist	2
Vicks® Sinex® VapoSpray™ 4-Hour	2
Vicks® Sinex® VapoSpray™ Moisturizing 12-Hour Decongestant UltraFine Mist	2
Vicks® VapoSyrup™ Severe Congestion Head & Chest Congestion Relief	2
Vivarin Caffeine Alertness Aid	14
Walgreens® Assorted Fruit Extra 750 mg Antacid Chewable Tablets	7
Walgreens® Extra Strength Antacid Tablets	7
Walgreens® Low Dose Aspirin Safety Coated Tablets	10
Walgreens® Maximum Strength Acid Controller Tablets	7
Walgreens® Menstrual Relief Aspirin Free Caplets Maximum Strength	8
Walgreens® Omeprazole Acid Reducer	7
Walgreens® WAL-ITIN® Indoor and Outdoor Allergy 24 Hour Relief	1
Walgreens® Wal-Zyr™ All Day Allergy Tablets	1
XL-3® Cold Medicine Tablets	1, 2
Zantac® Ranitidine Tablets 150 Mg Maximum Strength Acid Reducer	7
Zantac® Ranitidine Tablets 75 Mg Acid Reducer	7
Zegerid OTC Capsules	7
Zicam® Cough Max Cough Melts	2

(*continued*)

OTC Drug Name	Section(s)
Zicam® Cough Max Cough Spray	2
Zicam® Multi-Symptom Cold & Flu Daytime To Go	2
Zicam® Multi-Symptom Cold & Flu Liquid Daytime	2
Zicam® Multi-Symptom Cold & Flu Nighttime Liquid	2
Zicam® Multi-Symptom Cold & Flu Nighttime To Go	2
Zyrtec® 10 mg Liquid Gels	1
Zyrtec® Itchy Eye Drops	1
Zyrtec® Tablets	1
Zyrtec-D®	1